CHARLES VAN RIPER, editor ***Foundations of Speech Pathology Series***

| | |
|---|---|
| MARTHA BLACK | ***Speech Correction in the Schools*** |
| McKENZIE BUCK | ***Aphasia*** |
| JAMES A. CARRELL | ***Disorders of Articulation*** |
| FRED M. CHREIST | ***Foreign Accent*** |
| FREDERIC L. DARLEY | ***Diagnosis and Appraisal of Communication Disorders*** |
| LOUIS M. DI CARLO | ***The Deaf*** |
| EUGENE T. McDONALD<br>BURTON CHANCE | ***Cerebral Palsy*** |
| G. PAUL MOORE | ***Organic Voice Disorders*** |
| ALBERT MURPHY | ***Functional Voice Disorders*** |
| JOHN J. O'NEILL | ***The Hard of Hearing*** |
| FRANK B. ROBINSON | ***Introduction to Stuttering*** |
| DESO A. WEISS | ***Cluttering*** |
| HAROLD WESTLAKE<br>DAVID RUTHERFORD | ***Cleft Palate*** |
| NANCY E. WOOD | ***Delayed Speech and Language Development*** |

*Prentice-Hall Foundations of Speech Pathology Series*

PRENTICE-HALL INTERNATIONAL, INC., *London*
PRENTICE-HALL OF AUSTRALIA, PTY., LTD., *Sydney*
PRENTICE-HALL OF CANADA, LTD., *Toronto*
PRENTICE-HALL OF INDIA (PRIVATE) LTD., *New Delhi*
PRENTICE-HALL OF JAPAN, INC., *Tokyo*
PRENTICE-HALL DE MEXICO, S.A., *Mexico City*

***Introduction to Stuttering***

# *Introduction to Stuttering*

**Frank B. Robinson**

*Professor of Speech*
*and Director, Speech and Hearing Clinic*
*Miami University, Oxford, Ohio*

Prentice-Hall, Inc., *Englewood Cliffs, N. J.*

Library of Congress Catalog Card No.: 64-25204

Printed in the United States of America
49861-C

# editor's note

THE SET OF VOLUMES WHICH CONSTITUTES THE *Foundations of Speech Pathology* is designed to serve as the nucleus of a professional library, both for students of speech pathology and audiology and for the practicing clinician. Each individual text in the series is written by an author whose authority has long been recognized in his field. Each author has done his utmost to provide the basic information concerning the speech or hearing disorders covered in his book. Our new profession needs new tools, good ones, to be used not once but many times. The flood of new information already upon us requires organization if it is to be assimilated and if it is to help us solve the many different professional problems which beset us. This series provides that essential organization.

One of the unifying and outstanding features of all the volumes in this series is the use of search items. In addition to providing the core of information concerning his subject, each author has indicated clearly other sources having significance for the topic being discussed. The reader is urged to explore, to search, and to discover—and the trails are charted. In so rapidly changing a profession as ours, we cannot afford to remain content with what we have been taught. We must learn to continue learning.

Although each individual volume in this series is complete unto itself, the instructor should welcome the opportunity presented by the *Foundations of Speech Pathology* to combine several volumes to form the basic structure of the course he teaches. They may also be used as collateral readings. These short but comprehensive books give the instructor a thoroughly flexible teaching tool. But the primary aim of the authors of these texts has been the creation of a basic library for all of our students and professional workers. In this series we have sought to provide a common fund of knowledge to help unify and serve our new profession.

# *preface*

Among the several disorders the student of speech pathology is expected to understand, none creates confusion, frustration, and discouragement more frequently or with greater impact than stuttering. The disorder is explained in many different ways in many separate books. Much of the voluminous research is descriptive rather than explanatory. Courses devoted to the subject commonly offer either a thorough exposure to the instructor's preferred explanation or a broad coverage of many points of view with no imposed preference. Courses limited to a single point of view too often leave the student with a bias that makes it difficult to understand and/or accept any other possible explanations. Those that "cover the waterfront" tend to leave the student appalled by the length of the reading reference list and utterly confused about which explanation to adopt for practical purposes.

We know of no completely satisfactory solution. There is no simple, uncomplicated way to explain stuttering. There is no quick and painless way to acquire the available knowledge about this perplexing disorder of speech. We do, however, believe this book will make it somewhat easier for the student to obtain the basic information so essential for understanding the stutterers who will soon be coming to him for help.

The point of view of this book is this: Stuttering is revealed by a multiple number of differing combinations of attitudes and behavior patterns, it has its source in multiple conditions and/or circumstances, it tends to become a problem with multiple facets that vary greatly in their implications for treatment among individuals, and it responds best to multiple treatment approaches tailored to fit individual needs.

The book begins with descriptions of various patterns of behavior commonly found among those who stutter and a discussion of some of the puzzling features the stuttering frequently includes. Chapter 2 provides the reader with explanation of all the theories about the origin of stuttering that have been considered seriously during the twentieth century. Chapter 3 explains what is happening as early signs of stuttering change into more noticeable and troublesome forms of the disorder. Chapter 4 describes and explains the ultimate stage, secondary stuttering. Several cases are presented to illustrate how the problem which secondary stuttering represents varies among individuals and how the differences determine the kind or the emphasis of treatment. The concluding chapter returns the reader to stuttering in its earlier forms for a discussion of preventive measures. Illustrative cases again are used to demonstrate how specific approaches are related to individual needs.

Anyone expecting or possibly just hoping to find information about stuttering in this book that is sufficiently comprehensive will be disappointed. It is an introduction to the subject and no more than that. We have, however, tried to anticipate the reader's questions along the way. Carefully selected references have been inserted in the text throughout the book. They do not always lead to the only available answers and in some instances possibly not to the best ones. Nevertheless, we feel certain that those who read this book and study the references will not only be well prepared for advanced courses on the subject but will also find it easier to understand the stutterers they encounter.

I take this opportunity to express a debt of gratitude to Dr. Charles Van Riper for providing me with the opportunity to write this book and for being such a patient and considerate editor. I also wish to thank Mary Wagner and Gerrie Robinson for their valuable assistance.

F.B.R.

# contents

## chapter I



## chapter II

## chapter III



## chapter IV

***chapter V***

THE PROBLEM

UNDERSTANDING STUTTERING IS A FORMIDABLE TASK. THE student is challenged to comprehend a disorder which (*a*) is revealed by a perplexing variety of multiple behavior patterns, (*b*) is authoritatively explained in several different ways, and (*c*) responds with widely varying success to a host of treatments each of which generally is believed by its advocates to be the appropriate way to treat stutterers. In addition, the literature is so voluminous it is doubtful that anyone has read it all. And, finally, it seldom is possible for the student-in-training to obtain sufficient practical experience with stutterers before being confronted with full responsibility for their treatment as a

# 1 *the student's dilemma*

practicing therapist. Not an encouraging picture perhaps, but it would be grossly misleading to begin a book about stuttering for students of speech pathology by stating or implying that this disorder is easily understood. The complex nature of stuttering has defied precise explanation for centuries. Extensive research and clinical study, particularly during the past forty years, have revealed much about this disorder; but, like other human ills such as asthma, dermatitis, and the common cold, stuttering still contains mystery. Unfortunately, we cannot fold our hands and wait for complete explanation of this problem. Stutterers constitute approximately 1 per cent of each generation's population. They must have help now. Many come to speech therapists and, though it may not be possible yet for some time to provide satisfactory treatment or guidance for all, there is enough knowledge to protect many children from developing serious handicapping problems and to prevent others from being socially or economically handicapped by the difficulty. It is even possible to help some who have pronounced trouble to become completely free from stuttering. This knowledge must be acquired. The present book is planned to provide a fund of basic information about stuttering. It can serve only to begin a continuing study of this disorder. No single source will do the job. There are numerous other books to be read, journals and unpublished materials to be studied, and many actual stutterers to be explored.

### *Stuttering Behavior in the Young Child*

Suppose we begin by getting acquainted with the puzzling behavior patterns. They not only are multiple in form but markedly variant in frequency, severity, and complexity. People who stutter reveal the difficulty in many different ways. Perhaps it will help if we have you meet some like those you can expect to encounter.

> Here, for example, is an excerpt from a taped conversation with a four-year-old boy: "I . . . I . . . . . . . I went to . . . . . to to the suh . . . . suh . . . suh . . . suhcus (circus). We . . . we had our suh . . . suh . . . . . suh . . . suh . . suppuh (supper) theuh (there). The an . . . an . . . . animals an . . . animals all ate all . . . all they all ate too. It wuh . . wuh . . . was . . was fun."

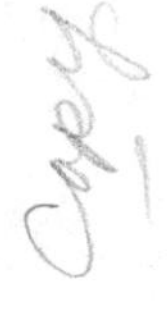

> Another youngster, a five-year-old boy, explains how a puzzle is assembled: "You . . . . . you . . . . . . . youput this piece here li . . . . . li . . . . . . li . . like . . . . . like this 'n then . . . . . . . n' then . . . . then this one well . . . . . well . . wellit goes it it goes well here see like li . . . . . . . li . . . . li . . . . like this."

Here we find the most frequent features of early stuttering. Fluency is disrupted by repetitions; sometimes of single words, sometimes of word elements, occasionally of word groups. However, there is more to these repetitions than can be illustrated on the printed page. They do not occur, for example, in as regular a rhythmic pattern as the illustrations suggest. The time between repetitions varies, creating an intermittent, hesitant quality in the speech. Then, too, some of the repetitions of the boy in the second sample were produced with heightened tension in the oral area. It was as though he had to force a bit to say such words as *you, well,* and *like.* Also, words may be linked together like *youput* and *wellit* in that same example. Frequently, when words are combined in this manner, the last sound of the first word will be prolonged.

In some youngsters, prolongation rather than repetition is the prominent feature of early symptoms.

> Here is an illustrative excerpt from an observation session with a three-year-old: "I . . . . . . . I-I-I-I-I . . . . . I don' wanna play-ay-ay-ay that . . . that game. Caaaaaaaaaan we may . . . . make soooome more p-pictures?"

Here, too, there was a slight strained quality of voice during the prolongations that isn't evident in a typed version. This additional dimension can be observed often in other children whose early stuttering includes similar prolongations.

> Still another common pattern is illustrated by the response of a five-year-old girl to a query about her favorite TV program. "The b . . . (here her lips became tightly pressed together for a brief time and then the first part of the desired word sort of exploded out of her mouth as 'beh.' Then again her lips became tightly locked in an exaggerated tension-posture on the *b*. After a release that brought forth another

'beh' followed once again by tightly pressed lips postured for the *b*, the complete word was exploded out of her mouth) best one is . . . is . . . . . . . . . . (now there was silence. Her mouth was open and she appeared to be struggling though there were no obvious signs of tension as there were for *best*. She then closed her mouth, said *is* again twice and then preceded the next word with a couple of 'uhs') uh . . . uh . . . Uncle Al." *Uncle* seemed very difficult for her to produce.

This obviously was more severe stuttering. Such difficulty can be painful to watch and we can appreciate the distress and frustration that must be experienced by such a speaker. And, indeed, unlike the children in the previous illustrations, this young stutterer was highly aware and concerned about her trouble. The mother reported that tears would begin to spill occasionally after a severe struggle on some word and the girl sometimes would momentarily refuse to talk after such an experience.

Such evident feelings of frustration and/or embarrassment are highly significant features of the disorder of stuttering. Speech pathologists generally agree that these feelings are responsible for most if not all of the speech disruptions and associated problems encountered among older children and adults. These features of the disorder will be discussed and amplified in later sections of this book. The task at this time is merely to become acquainted with some of the ways in which stuttering is revealed. Several of the common patterns found in the early stuttering of young children have been presented. We have seen how they vary from relatively uncomplicated repetitions to pronounced struggling utterance. They are not *always* as vivid or as frequent as we have illustrated in

1 O. Bloodstein, "The Development of Stuttering: 1. Changes in Nine Basic Features," *Journal of Speech and Hearing Disorders*, XXV

(1960), 219-34.
What other behavior patterns are reported among young stutterers in this study of 418 cases?

these few brief samples. Within a group of children and even in the same child, much variability may occur. Stuttering is an intermittent disorder. It comes and goes, especially in children. Periods of stuttering are interspersed between periods of fluency. And, even during the periods of stuttering, the difficulty varies. No child consistently stutters or stutters consistently.

### *An Initial Challenge*

Unusual forms or amounts of stuttering are easy to recognize, but the behavior in many young children looks and sounds very much like normal speech. Since all children fumble, hesitate, and repeat while learning to talk, parents and teachers often cannot be certain whether such disruptions are normal or abnormal. Speech therapists frequently must make the decision for them. We must begin early to train our eyes and ears. Every clinic has tapes which usually are available to the interested and responsible student. There are published films to be viewed, not once but many times. Also, most public-school therapists welcome occasional visits by students, and elementary-school teachers may permit student visitors to observe the recitations of young stutterers. The child who will be your first stuttering case is already born and you'll need to know much more than you can learn from the basic requirements of a three-credit hour course on the subject.

### *Behavior in the Older Stutterer: Overt Patterns*

Stuttering encountered in older children and adults is revealed by an even greater variety of behavior patterns.

Stuttering doesn't remain static. It grows. The disruptions in fluency tend to become more noticeable as well as more frequent. New ways of stuttering emerge to replace or embellish earlier ones. Whole new complicated patterns may be added. Early patterns of childhood may still appear, but stuttering in many older individuals bears little resemblance to beginning forms. Most obvious are changes in the visible and audible, or *overt,* behavior.

> One parent described developments in a ten-year-old boy this way: "For a long time when he was younger he just repeated a lot. We were concerned but were told not to pay any attention to it and not to have him treated for the difficulty. And it did go away. We hadn't seen any stuttering for over a year. Then, just about a year ago, he began having trouble again but not in the same way. It was terrible at times when he tried to talk. He'd squeeze his eyes and grit his teeth and sometimes he'd hit his fist against his leg. We didn't know what to do so we did nothing. It isn't so bad now, but then he isn't as talkative as he used to be either. He tells us it doesn't bother him and he didn't want any help for it, but we figured he just couldn't admit that he was upset. He refused to come with us to see you and we both wonder if it was the wrong thing to do."

Such accounts of advanced forms of stuttering by no means are unusual, though the change tends to be more gradual than was reported for this boy. Many other overt visible patterns may be noted among these older cases. Some include pronounced tremors of the lips, jaw, or tongue. Sometimes the tongue is literally protruded during moments of stuttering. Rigid postures of the head may occur. Facial grimaces and pronounced tension-postures of lips and tongue are quite common. Extraneous convulsive-like movements of the head or limbs may be observed. One adult of our acquaintance suddenly would look as though she were about to pray as she talked. Both palms would be placed together in front of her, pressed together tightly, then a word or phrase would be produced as she suddenly pulled them apart. Another moved her feet around as she talked. If she were standing, it would at times look like she were about to perform a soft-shoe routine. She had been mercilessly teased for years about this mannerism but had been unable to stop it from occurring whenever she had trouble talking. It had become an integral part of her stuttering behavior.

Overt patterns in the advanced stages of stuttering also may include various audible elements. Finger snapping, gasping or choking sounds, and exaggerated series of "uhs," "wells," or "and-uhs" are among those found in the stuttering patterns of these people. Sometimes odd noises accompany the head postures or extraneous movements. One of our cases, a twenty-five-year-old man, would pause before some words and gulp noisily, at least twice, before attempting the desired words. Gulping audibly takes considerable time as well as coordination in the middle of a sentence. And it is laughably absurd to some listeners. It shouldn't be difficult to understand why this man seldom talked, never had been on a real date, and had reconciled himself to a solitary life on a secluded farm. Another audible pattern found among older stutterers involves excessive prolonging of sounds.

> Here's the way one seventh-grade boy told us about his difficulty: "I just s-s-s-s-s-s-seem to get s-s-s-s-s (here he stopped, inhaled, and started over) s-s-s-s-stuck on that . . . . .-s-s-s-s-sound." He often expelled practically all air from his lungs before completing troublesome words and at times, as on *stuck*, he would interrupt the prolongation to take in more air. This boy had similar though less pronounced trouble on the [f] and [sh] sounds as well as tonic-type blocks on plosive consonants. But *s* words caused him the

most trouble. He said he often wished someone would invent an English language that didn't have that sound.

### *Covert Patterns*

The peculiarity and variety of overt behavior patterns are two of the more puzzling features of stuttering. However, among older stutterers, there are other patterns which often are more difficult to recognize and comprehend. These are the many forms of covert behavior associated with the disorder. Some stutterers seldom if ever exhibit behavior that directly or obviously indicates their stuttering problem. They hide it. They detour around expected trouble. They filibuster with words they can say fluently. They work to avoid situations in which stuttering is anticipated. As long as they succeed in the avoiding or the disguise behavior, the stuttering may not be observable.

A college freshman with this general type of stuttering pattern reported: "Very few kids in my high school knew I stuttered. We moved to this town when I was a sophomore and I just acted like I wasn't much of a talker. I had lots of friends and went almost everywhere with them. Most of the time I got along all right by letting someone else order stuff like tickets or hamburgs or I'd just take the same thing somebody else got. For awhile it was awful hard. I was in a constant sweat. But after awhile I'd picked up a lot of tricks and things were pretty easy. When I got stuck and really stuttered, I often would start coughing like I had a cold or something. I can't say I was real happy in high school but I wasn't miserable either. I went with one girl all during my junior year and she never knew I stuttered. But here in college it's been different. My old tricks don't seem to work. Besides, I want to get into a fraternity and I hate to play a lie with those fellows. So I finally decided to get some help."

Here we find the stuttering hidden behind a camouflage

of tricks. You will encounter many stutterers similar to this young man, though usually they won't come so willingly for help. These people hate their stuttering. They will deny its existence. They may refuse to cooperate in any treatment plan. Those who do seek help frequently confound inexperienced therapists by proceeding to sabotage their sincere efforts to help. When the tricks can be exposed in these cases, severe overt stuttering often appears. We must understand this common result of therapy with such cases and acquire skill in helping them come to grips with their problem. Yet, in other instances, removing the tricks results in almost complete fluency. These stutterers find that the thing they feared and hated doesn't materialize at all on most expected occasions and the slight disruptions that do occur may indeed be surprisingly tolerable. Whatever it was that caused them to acquire all the covert behavior no longer happens! Relief erases fear and they improve rapidly. Many patterns of stuttering are indeed extraordinary and full of mysteries.

#### *Consistency of Stuttering Behavior*

Variability in frequency and severity, as well as puzzling inconsistencies, also characterize stuttering *in each individual.* Every stutterer experiences perplexing fluctuations in difficulty from week to week, day to day, from situation to situation. Predicted trouble may not materialize. Anticipated freedom from stuttering in a particular situation may turn into a nightmare of broken speech.

> One adult male felt this was the worst feature of the problem: "Sometimes I think I would rather be blind or missing a leg than have this damn stuttering. At least then I would always know I was going to have certain kinds of trouble. The way it is with this stuff is maddening. I never can be

really sure. Except maybe when I sing or get mad. I don't remember ever stuttering at those times. I sang in a quartet and in the high-school glee club, and about the other, it used to be quite a joke among my friends. They'd say, 'Just get ol' George mad and then he can talk up a storm.' "

Such inconsistencies are universal with stutterers but are not the same for every individual. It is generally believed that all are fluent when singing and it does seem to be true for the majority. However, we have tape recordings of two people who reveal considerable stuttering in their singing and most speech therapists occasionally encounter others with similar histories. Reading aloud causes some stutterers to have great trouble, more than they usually have when just talking; others can speak fluently from the printed page. Some stutter more when talking to people within their own general age bracket or of the same sex; others have little or no trouble in such circumstances but stutter wretchedly around older people or those of the opposite sex. We knew one severe stutterer who seldom had any trouble whenever he talked to fat male adults but never experienced the same degree of fluency if the audience were females of similar proportions. Many stutterers claim that a few drinks will free their tongues as it does for most nonstutterers yet others report that alcohol causes them to stutter more.

In summary, stuttering or stammering is revealed in

2 We consider these terms synonymous, as do most other speech pathologists in this country. For information about an exception to this point of view, read C. S. Bluemel, *The Riddle of Stuttering* (Danville, Illinois: The Interstate Printers & Publishers, Inc., 1957), pp. 7-10.

many different ways and has proved to be a difficult disorder to define. Nine leading authorities (*8*) recently sum-

3 Compare definitions of stuttering from the following sources:

M. Solomon, "Stuttering as an Emotional and Personality Disorder," *Journal of Speech Disorders,* IV (1939), 347.

I. P. Glauber, "The Psychoanalysis of Stuttering," in *Stuttering: A Symposium,* ed. S. Eisenson (New York: Harper & Row, Publishers, Inc., 1958), p. 78.

W. Johnson, *Speech Handicapped School Children* (New York: Harper & Row, Publishers, Inc., 1956), p. 217.

L. Travis, *Handbook of Speech Pathology* (New York: Appleton-Century-Crofts, Inc., 1957), p. 919.

B. Bryngelson, "Theoretic and Therapeutic Considerations of Dysphemia and Its Symptom, Stuttering," in *Stuttering: Significant Theories and Therapies,* ed. E. F. Hahn (Stanford University: Stanford University Press, 1947), p. 19.

C. Van Riper, *Speech Correction: Principles and Methods,* 4th ed. (Englewood Cliffs, N. J., Prentice-Hall, Inc., 1963), p. 311.

R. West, M. Ansberry, and A. Carr, *The Rehabilitation of Speech* (New York: Harper & Row, Publishers, Inc., 1957), p. 15.

J. Sheehan, "Conflict Theory of Stuttering," in *Stuttering: A Symposium,* ed. J. Eisenson (New York: Harper & Row, Publishers, Inc., 1958), p. 123.

marized their opinions on the multiple features of the disorder by listing six separate characteristics by which stuttering may be revealed:

1. Facial contortions, blockings, strugglings, prolongations, breaks in rhythm of speech, or other signs of breakdown in the forward flow of speech to a degree that sets the speaker off from his associates.
2. An understanding between speaker and listener that stuttering actually has taken place—that is, that the speaker is trying to speak without these interferences, but often fails in the attempt.
3. Some feelings of frustration and helplessness brought on by the difficulties plus the fear of possible difficulty.
4. Some feelings of fearfulness or concern about the ability to speak at all.
5. Anxiety concerning uncertainties—not necessarily connected with speaking—and which interferes with speaking ability.
6. The speaker having a picture of himself as a stutterer,

perhaps a troubled awareness that his way of talking is unnatural and is disturbing to the listener.

It appears that stuttering is as difficult to define as intelligence or humor. Any single term seems inadequate for such a collection of distinguishing features. Perhaps several separate terms would make more sense even though common elements are found among all stutterers. However, at the present time, certain patterns of behavior generally are recognized in our society as stuttering by both the speaker and his listener and it is with these that the quest for knowledge about stuttering always begins.

LET'S BEGIN AT THE BEGINNING. STUTTERING USUALLY HAS ITS onset some time during the preschool years, frequently between the ages of two and four. When it begins in later life, and particularly in the adult years, its source can usually be traced to emotional trauma or central nervous system damage. Its beginnings in young children are much more difficult to explain. Great controversy exists about the identification and origin of the early behavior. Is it, as some claim, identical to the broken speech commonly found in all other children at times? Is it no more than a reflection of universal difficulties encountered in learning to talk or developing in other ways? Are stutterers simply

# 2 sources of beginning stuttering

the few unfortunates who happen to encounter unique "climates" that impose the disorder on normal organisms? Or does the broken speech of some children differ in amount and/or form and thus suggest a special seed, so to speak, for stuttering? In short, can the beginnings of stuttering be explained as normal behavior or do they reveal the effects of a deviant organism?

## Early concepts

(Statements about etiology, prior to the present century, generally reflected the belief that all stuttering represented one and the same problem and revealed the effects of some singular condition. In Roman times, for example, stutterers were viewed as being possessed by evil spirits. During the

Middle Ages, it was commonly thought that stutterers' tongues were somehow inadequate for the fluency demands of speech. Variations of this particular idea persisted for centuries. Treatments to overcome some presumed organic or functional fault of that structure were still being utilized late in the nineteenth century and such practices may be found occasionally even today. As recently as 1957, for example, patent number 2,818,065 was issued for the FREED STAMMERCHECK, an oral appliance designed to slow tongue movement and thus assist in the reduction of stammering (stuttering) symptoms. The patent account (9) states, "When the device is properly fitted in the mouth of a stutterer an immediate improvement in his speech has been observed, and with only intermittent wearing, the reflex habit has been broken."

Historical accounts of stuttering include several other structures whose faulty size, shape, or operation was thought to be the basic factor. According to Klingbeil (*18:*115-32), the disorder has been attributed by various authors to such different parts as the hyoid bone, the larynx, the palatal arch, the lips, and the pharynx. Others believed that stuttering was due to some central nerve derangement, that it was a special form of chorea, that it was caused by mental debility, by faulty action of the respiratory muscles, or that it simply was a bad habit. During the latter half of the nineteenth century, some workers began to view stuttering as a neurosis and psychoanalysts claimed it was a form of hysteria, with its neurotic core in traumatic early childhood experiences.

Also, during the latter half of the nineteenth century, we began to find information suggesting that the more pronounced and bizarre patterns of stuttering represent a separate aspect of the problem. Klencke (*17*) suggested such a distinction in 1862. He believed those revealed the stutterer's attempts to avoid or release himself from some basic inability to utter syllables. Later, Ssikorski (*29*) and Wyllie (*42*) offered additional support for the idea that stuttering behavior varies according to the course of the disorder. Then we find Froeschels (*11*:1109-11), writing in the early years of the present century, referring to early repetitions as *primary clonus,* subsequent tense prolongations as *tonus,* and considering all other associated behavior a result of emotional reactions to occurrences of the two basic forms. And at about the same time Bluemel (*5*:91-102) introduced the terms *primary* and *secondary* to indicate the perceived distinction between characteristic beginning signs of stuttering, believed to be caused by some fundamental difficulty, and later behavior created by the stutterer's emotionally bound struggles with the primary forms of trouble.

The concept of stuttering as a multiple phase, or stage, disorder was widely accepted. Although seriously challenged by Johnson's semantically oriented viewpoint introduced in the 1930's, Bluemel's terms became firmly established among speech pathologists in this country and profoundly influenced treatment methods. Primary stutterers were considered to need a distinctly different form of treatment from those who presented secondary patterns. It is only within recent years that certain accumulated information has again challenged the dichotomous classification. This time it is in the direction of additional categories and we shall have more to say about this development in a later section. At the moment, we are concerned only with pointing out that stuttering no longer is viewed generally as one and the same kind of problem throughout its course in each and every individual.

Ideas about the basic cause of stuttering have been characterized for centuries by (*a*) belief in some single etiological factor and (*b*) great variance in opinions about what the factor is. Modern literature continues to reflect

4 For information about early beliefs that begins with Herodotus some 400 years B.C. and ends with Coriat in 1915, read the historical account referred to earlier by Klingbeil (p. 14).

Then, for viewpoints of twenty-five twentieth-century workers, read E. F. Hahn, *Stuttering: Significant Theories and Therapies* (Stanford University: Stanford University Press, 1943).

How many different causes of stuttering are claimed by contributors to this latter reference? Who besides Weiss postulates more than a single cause?

marked disagreement on the question of the underlying cause. This is true despite the fact that stuttering for the past three decades has been the target of more research and clinical study than any other disorder of speech. Thousands of pages by dedicated scholars have been written to explain and support innumerable ideas. Individuals have arrived at their own conclusions and most can provide vigorous and logical defenses for their views. However, none has been able to satisfactorily substantiate a solitary origin for all cases except in theory. Therapists who attempt to treat stuttering believing it to have a single cause soon encounter puzzling exceptions which refuse to fit into the solitary concept. If some singular condition responsible for the beginning of stuttering in every instance does exist, it has succeeded in remaining hidden from view. West (*40*:169) has succinctly summarized the situation by stating: "It is interesting to me that in the 30 years my name has been on the roles of the American Speech and Hearing Association the percentage of membership who profess to know the precise etiology of stuttering has steadily fallen."

### *Why?*

Why should it prove so difficult to isolate and identify the origin of stuttering? What is there about this particular human ailment that makes its source such a phantom? The

answers seem to lie partly in the complex nature of oral communication and partly in the gradual and insidious manner in which stuttering usually begins.

Oral communication is an elaborately complicated facet of human behavior. It may be said to have two major aspects, the *speech process* and the *speech act*. The process includes the speaker's concepts, his language system, his intent (of which at times he may be only vaguely aware and on occasion completely unaware), and the complex interrelationships between speaker and listener. The speech act refers to the relatively mechanical production of words. Its basic components include the neurological, structural, and muscle systems involved in word production plus various sensory feedback systems essential for monitoring the performance. Both process and act are acquired gradually through maturation and learning and both in time tend to function more or less automatically in most situations.

This is especially true for the speech act. The act of speaking is servant to the process of communication. Moreover, it has its rate and style dictated by the culture. Individual words generally must be uttered speedily as well as accurately. Each sound and syllable in a word must be succeeded almost immediately by the next. So, too, must each word in a phrase or sentence unit. Hence, patterns for the speech act must become firmly established so that the mouth can perform much like a robot. Words must flow in an automated manner, with incredibly fast checking and correction devices to maintain the required standards.

5 For some background information on this aspect of talking, see R. West, "The Neurophysiology of Speech," in *Handbook of Speech Pathology*, ed. L. Travis (New York: Appleton-Century-Crofts, 1957), Chapter 3, and C. Van Riper and J. Irwin, *Voice and Articulation* (Englewood Cliffs, N. J.: Prentice-Hall, Inc., 1958), Chapter 6.

The amalgamation of process and act for normal oral-communication skill demands of the human organism the individual integrity and precise coordination of many systems. As Berry and Eisenson (*3:*40) say, "We speak with the entire body—nerves, muscles, glands, and blood. All must enter into superb integrations, which are in turn correlated with past learning. No human activity, perhaps, requires greater coordination than speech." Thus, when a speaker falters, when breaks in the automaticity of the act are revealed by disruptions in fluency, the identification of a specific responsible agent becomes a redoubtable task.

Equally troublesome problems occur in any search for the origin of stuttering because of the manner in which it is first revealed. Beginning signs tend to be mild and transient. They appear only infrequently as brief sieges of repetitions or prolongations, interspersed by periods of fluency that may last for weeks or months or, on occasion, for years, as Bloodstein (*4:*225) found. Even when the earliest signs are severe in form or excessive in amount, they still come and go, and the intervening periods of fluency serve to dissipate any parental concern. Few parents become sufficiently worried to make their children available for professional observations and evaluations until long after the first signs were noted. By this time, the underlying cause may be obscured by the factors which operated to precipitate the change that motivated the parent to seek advice. Investigators now must rely on memories. Most parents understandably have great difficulty recalling the earliest instances of broken speech. Also, many parents aren't particularly accurate in reporting other events in their children's early lives. Thus, it

6 E. A. Haggard, A. Brekstad, and A. G. Skard, "On the Reliability of the Amamnestic Interview," *Journal of Abnormal and Social Psychology,* LXI (1960), 311-18.

Which of the following statements are supported by results or conclusions of this study?

1. The presence of anxiety in mothers during early experiences with their children tends to cause them to forget the experience.
2. Mothers do not remember early experiences of their children with any greater accuracy than fathers.
3. If a mother's memory is reliable for first-year events in her child's life, it will be dependabe for information about later years.

becomes important to have subjects to study when signs of the disorder first appear.

This presents several problems. The most critical, already alluded to, is the difficulty in accurate identification of early stuttering. When can it be said that the occurrence of disruptions in a child's speech indicate or presage a genuine disorder of fluency? This question has been the crux of a major controversy among speech pathologists for some thirty years. Some believe the collected evidence clearly indicates that early occurrences of broken speech are rarely anything but normal behavior. Others believe there are certain differences in the early fluency disruptions of some children which justify their consideration as something other than normal. The issue remains unresolved, and, even though investigators might be prepared to administer tests that possibly could reveal some causative agent, there no doubt would be violent disagreement about when to tell parents to bring their children in for such research purposes.

One logical approach is the longitudinal-type study. Children would be followed from birth or early infancy through the first three or four years, with investigators periodically collecting samples of fluency disruptions along with information from tests, observations, medical records, and questioning of parents. Then, when stuttering became clearly obvious, information would be available that might disclose distinguishing features of the early disruptions as well as some common condition or experience.

However, we must remember that stuttering occurs only in about 1 per cent of the population. And, though it does appear repeatedly in certain families in some apparently inheritable manner, its occurrence even in those instances can't be predicted accurately for any particular newborn child. The many problems able to be envisioned in a longitudinal study of sufficient numbers of children for information on the few who would turn out to be stutterers probably explains why the approach hasn't been utilized.

### The current situation

The fact that beginning stuttering is so difficult to research may mean it will be some time yet before its precise etiology becomes known. Meanwhile, even though therapists discover that treatment limited to the troublesome speech behavior is all some stutterers seem to require, it is highly important for the student to acquire a working concept about basic etiology. The results of treatments based on attention to the stuttering behavior alone tend to be impermanent. Stutterers so treated must often seek help again. And, for some, it becomes again and again. Parents who become concerned about signs of beginning stuttering come to the speech therapist expecting at least to have the difficulty explained and most want to be told what to do about it. Clinical consideration of underlying factors is a must for effective work with these parents and their children as well as for helping older stutterers achieve solutions that last.

The present state of our knowledge means that counseling and treatment procedures must rest more or less precariously on assumptions about etiology. Current literature and professional practices offer a choice between three general suppositions.

1. *Stuttering has its origin in a singular condition or circumstance.* This is the traditional point of view and some modern therapists continue to believe in its greater validity.

2. *The origin of stuttering is still a complete mystery; it is useless to assume a particular etiology or to search for one from examination or case-history material.* Treatment in accordance with this point of view is aimed at alleviating or possibly eliminating those factors that presently appear to be maintaining or aggravating the stuttering behavior.

3. *Stuttering has multiple origins.* Advocates of this belief claim the source of stuttering may be different for individuals. Identification of the underlying cause with absolute confidence seldom is considered possible. Thus, treatment must be initiated on the basis of a tentative conclusion about the most probable cause among several possibilities.

We find stuttering being treated effectively today from all three viewpoints. However, there appears to be a distinct trend among speech pathologists in this country toward the concept of multiple etiologies. Beginning stuttering is being viewed by an increasing number of workers as an indication of disruption or breakdown in fluency that represents the effects of various separate conditions or circumstances in different cases. Also, according to Bluemel

7 O. Bloodstein, "Stuttering as an Anticipatory Struggle Reaction," p. 12; J. Sheehan, "Conflict Theory of Stuttering," p. 136; J. Eisenson, "A Perseverative Theory of Stuttering," pp. 250, 255; and C. Van Riper, "Experiments in Stuttering Therapy," p. 390—all in *Stuttering: A Symposium*, ed. J. Eisenson (New York: Harper & Row, Publishers, Inc., 1958).

W. Johnson, *et al.*, *Speech Handicapped School Children*, Rev Ed.

(New York: Harper & Row, Publishers, Inc., 1956), pp. 263-64.
C. Bluemel, *The Riddle of Stuttering* (Danville, Ill.: The Interstate Printers & Publishers, Inc.), pp. 21-45.

Find a specific supporting statement for multiple etiology in each of these references. What additional support or contrary evidence can you find for the concept of multiple etiologies in more recently published books or current issues of professional journals?

(*6*:32), beginning signs of the disorder in individual cases may reflect different sources on separate occasions.

Our personal bias is doubtless apparent. The concept of multiple etiologies, to us, is the most sensible point of view at the present time. We believe it makes it possible to provide more appropriate advice to parents and more effective help for stutterers. In our clinical experience we have entories to permit us to accept the idea of a single cause. And countered too many stutterers with too many different histoo many also have been encountered for whom a specific underlying cause was too clear and too obvious to let us feel that treatment can never reflect basic etiology. At the same time, we must confess in all honesty that there have been a few children with whom we have failed to prevent the development of advanced stuttering behavior even though the "obvious" cause was successfully eliminated, or so we thought.

## THE POSSIBLE SOURCES

We now present a list of theories about the origin of stuttering that have been considered seriously during the twentieth century. Some are supported by results from experimental research, others by the weight of comparison with problems considered analogous to stuttering. A few haven't yet passed much beyond the speculative stage. Some will seem more logical. Some may make little sense. We make no special case for any, though some are easier to relate to actual instances of the disorder. We believe it is important that the professional speech therapist become familiar with all.

## Cerebral dominance and dysphemia

One group of ideas shares the premise that beginning stuttering is associated with some fundamental constitutional difference of kind or degree. Two of the earliest of this group to be seriously considered by speech pathologists in this country were the theories of cerebral dominance and dysphemia.

### *Cerebral Dominance*

The basic concept of this theory was developed by Orton (*25*) in connection with reading, writing, and speech problems in general. It was applied to stuttering by Travis during the late 1920's and popularized within the profession through his first text (*36*). The essential element of this concept of cerebral dominance in connection with stuttering is related to the precise coordinations of many paired muscle groups which are innervated from different sides of the brain during the act of talking. Thus, to move the tongue for speech purposes, impulses must be initiated from both cortical hemispheres and then arrive simultaneously at nerve endings in muscles on both sides of that important oral structure. This demands an integration of activities between the two hemispheres which was hypothesized as possible only if one of them was functionally dominant, serving as a master control unit, so to speak. It was thought that the majority of stutterers were people who lacked sufficient margins of unilateral dominance for proper coordination under all circumstances. If the margin were small (equilateral), stuttering would be triggered by relatively small amounts of stress, such as physical fatigue or emotional upset. As the margin approximated unilateral dominance, the individual was presumed to be less and less vulnerable to the triggering or precipitating conditions. In some cases, the confused laterality was believed due to an inherited system incapable of providing satisfactory unilateral motor leads for speech. Others acquired stuttering when the normal development of unilateral dominance was disrupted by certain environmental influences, such as the forced changing of handedness.

Support for the theory was claimed from results of studies of behavior associated with moments of stuttering, voluntary rhythmical movements of such structures as the tongue, lips, and diaphragm dissociated with speech, studies of writing and handedness, and subsequently of brain waves.

8 For an extensive account of the theory and related early research read L. Travis, *Speech Pathology* (New York: Appleton-Century-Crofts, Inc., 1931).

What additional support is offered by these later studies?

B. Bryngelson, "Sidedness as an Etiological Factor in Stuttering," *Journal of Genetic Psychology*, XLVII (1935), 204-17.

B. Bryngelson and B. Rutherford, "A Comparative Study of Laterality of Stutterers and Non-stutterers," *Journal of Speech Disorders*, II (1937), 15-16.

C. Van Riper, "The Quantitative Measurement of Laterality," *Journal of Experimental Psychology*, XVIII (1935), 372-82.

Y. Hunsley, "Disintegration in the Speech Musculature of Stutterers during the Production of a Non-vocal Temporal Pattern," *Psychological Monographs*, XLIX (1937), 32-49.

D. Lindsley, "Bilateral Differences in Brain Potentials from the Two Cerebral Hemispheres in Relation to Laterality and Stuttering," *Journal of Experimental Psychology*, XXVI (1940), 211-25.

N. Freestone, "A Brain-Wave Interpretation of Stuttering," *Quarterly Journal of Speech*, XXVIII (1942), 466-68.

L. Douglass, "A Study of Bilaterally Recorded Electroencephalograms of Adult Stutterers," *Journal of Experimental Psychology*, XXXII (1943), 247-65.

R. Dew, "Electroencephalographic Study of Stutterers during Sleep," *Speech Monographs,* XXIX (1952), 192.

E. Froeschels, "Is Handedness Organic or Functional in Nature?" *American Journal of Psychotherapy,* XV (1961), 101-105.

### *Dysphemia*

The dysphemia theory was introduced into the literature on stuttering by West (*41*). He utilized the term, which literally means disturbed speech in Greek, to imply an inner condition for which stuttering is the observable manifestation. However, unlike the cerebral dominance theory, no precise etiologic referrent was specified. Instead, the responsible agent was defined broadly by West (*41*:60) as "a physiological condition of the human organism, which, though not markedly disturbing the basic functions of the muscles of the speech apparatus, seriously interferes with the learned uses of those same muscles, particularly when those uses are emotionally and socially motivated." Thus, stuttering is viewed as a reflection of some unspecified constitutional difference that affects the fluency of speech adversely under certain circumstances. West supported his theory in part by pointing out inescapable facts about the greater incidence of stuttering among males (who appear to reveal generally slower rates of neuromotor maturation) and the occurrence in some families of multiple instances of stuttering that cannot be explained satisfactorily by imitation or social learning. Additional evidence was claimed from studies of blood chemistry and metabolism and of certain motor skills.

9 What specific evidence to support the dysphemia theory is provided by the studies listed below? Which offer equally logical support for the cerebral dominance theory?

R. West, "A Neurological Test for Stutterers," *Journal of Neurology and Psychopathology,* X (1929), 114-18.

G. Kopp, "Metabolic Studies of Stutterers," *Speech Monographs,* I (1934), 117-34.

M. Seemann,"A Contribution to the Pathology of Stuttering," *Review of Neurology and Psychiatry,* XXXII (1935), 399-404.

M. Palmer and A. Gillett, "Sex Differences in the Cardiac Rhythms of Stutterers," *Journal of Speech Disorders,* III (1938), 3-12.

L. Travis, "Dissociation of the Homologous Muscle Function in Stuttering," *Archives of Neurology and Psychiatry,* XXXI (1934), 127-31.

S. Nelson, "The Role of Heredity in Stuttering," *Journal of Pediatrics,* XIV (1939), 642-56.

H. Kopp, "The Relationship of Stuttering to Motor Disturbances," *The Nervous Child,* II (1943), 107-16.

M. Snyder, "Stuttering and Coordination," *Logos,* I (1958), 36-44.

Both theories received ardent support among speech pathologists for several years. During the 1930's and early 1940's, most speech therapists routinely advised parents not to interfere with any child's tendency towards left-handedness lest the resulting cerebral imbalance initiate signs of stuttering. And therapy for individuals with established patterns of stuttering commonly included procedures for strengthening unilateral cortical motor leads. Those stutterers were then taught various control techniques for countering any remaining effects of the presumed underlying neurological anomaly.

However, enthusiasm for either of these theories as a universal explanation for stuttering has gradually waned. For every study with supporting evidence, another has offered inconclusive or contradictory results. The theories

10 Compare information in the following references with that from Nos. 8 and 9.

M. Steer, "Symptomatologies of Young Stutterers," *Journal of Speech Disorders,* II (1937), 3-13.

H. Scarborough, "A Quantitative and Qualitative Analysis of the Electroencephalograms of Stutterers and Non-stutterers," *Journal of Experimental Psychology,* XXXII (1943), 156-67.

E. Daniels, "An Analysis of the Relation between Handedness and Stuttering with Special Reference to the Orton-Travis Theory of Cerebral Dominance," *Journal of Speech Disorders,* V (1940), 309-26.

M. Gray, "The X Family: A Clinical and Laboratory Study of a 'Stuttering' Family," *Journal of Speech Disorders,* V (1940), 343-48.

P. Finkelstein and S. Weisberger, "The Motor Proficiency of Stutterers," *Journal of Speech and Hearing Disorders,* XIX (1954), 52-58.

D. Williams, "Masseter Muscle Action Potentials in Stuttered and Non-stuttered Speech," *Journal of Speech and Hearing Disorders,* XX (1955), 242-61.

F. S. Brodnitz, "Stuttering of Different Types in Identical Twins," *Journal of Speech and Hearing Disorders,* XVI (1951), 334-36.

R. McCroskey, "Effect of Speech on Metabolism: A Comparison between Stutterers and Non-stutterers," *Journal of Speech and Hearing Disorders,* XXII (1957), 46-52.

For critiques of these theories, see:

C. Bluemel, "The Dominant Gradient in Stuttering," *Quarterly Journal of Speech,* XIX (1933), 233-42.

H. Hill, "Stuttering: A Critical Review and Evaluation of Biochemical Investigations," *Journal of Speech Disorders,* IX (1944), 245-61.

H. Hill, "Stuttering: A Review of Integration of Physiological Data," *Journal of Speech Disorders,* IX (1944), 289-324.

E. Froeschels, "New Viewpoints on Stuttering," *Folia Phoniatrica,* XIII (1961), 187-201.

have proved impossible to verify, perhaps because their formulations made them invulnerable to crucial testing. Both ideas required accurate evidence of central nervous system activity associated with overt behavior. We know of no greater challenge to man's ingenuity, even today, than trying to specify what is occurring neurologically in a live human being while he is actively behaving.

11 Explore the exciting developments in this field as portrayed in W. Penfield and L. Roberts, *Speech and the Brain Mechanism* (Princeton, N. J.: Princeton University Press, 1959).

Despite the failure of research to validate the universal application of either of these theories, the idea of a constitutional explanation for the disorder has persisted. West in time modified his concept of dysphemia, but he has

12 What is West's present definition of dysphemia and its relationship to stuttering? See R. West, M. Ansberry, and A. Carr, *The Rehabilitation of Speech,* 3rd ed. (New York: Harper & Row, Publishers, 1957), pp. 15 and 269.

Compare with C. Van Riper, *Speech Correction,* 4th ed. (Englewood Cliffs, N. J.: Prentice-Hall, Inc., 1963), p. 324.

maintained his basic thesis that beginning stuttering is a reflection of some fundamental biologic variation from the norm. His most recent contribution (*40:* Chapter 4) pursues the idea with a discussion about the resemblance of many stuttering blocks to the minute seizures associated with pyknolepsy, a mild childhood form of epilepsy. He notes the momentary and intermittent characteristics common to both disorders and points out that early signs of stuttering frequently disappear spontaneously just as the symptoms of pyknolepsy typically are gone by the early teen years. He believes the information suggests some common or at least similar developmental abnormality (a transient imbalance of blood chemistry in cases of stuttering) that operates periodically to cause momentary neuromotor malfunctioning whenever the system is exposed to sufficient stress to trigger the breakdown.

13 The more inquisitive student may want to explore this interesting possibility. See W. Penfield and H. Jasper, *Epilepsy and the Functional Anatomy of the Human Brain* (Boston: Little-Brown & Co., 1954); F. Gibbs and F. Stamps, *Epilepsy Handbook* (Springfield, Ill: C. C. Thomas, 1958); J. Toman, "Physiological Triggering Mechanisms in Childhood Epilepsy," *American Journal of Orthopsychiatry,* XXXII (1962), 507-14.

Travis also continued to express his belief in an underlying constitutional factor, though he began to attach greater significance to precipitating influences, principally traumatic experiences in infancy and childhood (*35:*3-5). His most recent views on the subject show a decisive shift in that direction.

14 What is Travis' present point of view? See L. Travis, "The Unspeakable Feelings of People with Special Reference to Stuttering," in *Handbook of Speech Pathology,* ed. L. Travis (New York: Appleton-Century-Crofts, Inc., 1957), pp. 916-47.

Variations of the constitutional theme continue to be found in the theoretical constructs of numerous other modern authorities. Bluemel, for example, considers beginning stammering (stuttering) to be an indication of a genuine "speech-deficiency." He tells us (*6*:27): ". . . he (the stammerer) is handicapped in his fluency just as the tone-deaf person is handicapped in music and the color-blind person is handicapped in art." We find Karlin (*16*: 61-64) reiterating his earlier (*15*:319-22) psychosomatic point of view that "stuttering is basically due to a delay or to a slower progress of myelinization of the cortical association areas concerned with speech." An organic anomaly is indicated by Eisenson (*7*: Chapter 5) who, in explaining his theory of stuttering as a perseverative phenomenon, states: "A majority of stutterers (from 55 to 60 per cent) are predisposed to a manner of oral language behavior called stuttering because they are constitutionally inclined to perseverate to an extent or degree greater than is the case for most speakers."

Still another theory that postulates a constitutional basis for stuttering is offered by Weiss (*39*:216-28). He has long

15 For his most recent formulation, see Deso Weiss, *Cluttering*, Prentice-Hall Foundations of Speech Pathology Series (Englewood Cliffs, N. J.: Prentice-Hall, Inc., 1964).

felt that nearly all stuttering is an outgrowth of cluttering, and believes that both disorders are rooted in a basic deficiency of the language function. Freund (*10*:689-705) expresses a similar conviction about stutterers who have a background of cluttering, though he disagrees with Weiss about the proportion of cases for which the theory is applicable.

The absence of scientific proof for any of these theories cannot be denied. However, the cumulative theoretical evidence is impressive and we do not believe it should be ignored as long as cases are encountered like Russell.

Russell was a sixteen-year-old junior in high school who had stuttered since early childhood when he came to our attention. His stuttering consisted predominantly of noticeable tension-postures on such sounds as the [p], [b], [k], [g], [f], [v], and [dʒ] and frequently included tremors of the lips or lower jaw. He stuttered often, but the blocks were relatively brief and were consistent in form. Adaptation was negligible (he stuttered about as frequently on the third and fourth readings of the same paragraph of material as on the first). He had a good attitude about the trouble. He seldom avoided speaking situations or specific words. He had had some speech therapy in the second grade, and his mother told us it had helped his feelings of embarrassment about the difficulty a great deal, but that it seemed to have had little effect on the actual amount of stuttering. Personality questionnaires indicated good emotional stability and revealed other evidence of an emotionally healthy home environment. His academic record was good though he had a long history of difficulties with reading and spelling and was still having more trouble with courses demanding language than it seemed he should. He had begun to learn typing because so many of his teachers complained about his hand-written papers.

Other notable items included: (*a*) ambidexterity—he wrote right-handed, but threw and sometimes reached for things with his left, (*b*) a history of early difficulties with writing that included a persistent tendency for reversals, (*c*) his father and a paternal uncle were left-handed and both had histories of stuttering (the father reported his speech difficulty had disappeared by the fourth or fifth grade, but that his brother still showed signs of stuttering), and (*d*) a pronounced tendency for more stuttering for a day or two after bad colds and other illnesses and when he was especially tired or excited.

We worked with Russell for two semesters. The basic approach consisted of teaching him to initiate troublesome words or syllables without the tremors and with a minimum of tension in the oral area. We also arranged for him to get some help for the spelling and English difficulties. He was extremely cooperative, did a lot of reading about stuttering on his own, and responded well to the treatment approach. The stuttering became markedly reduced in both frequency and severity, but his speech was still characterized by frequent "stickings" on initial plosives. Periodic reports were received through the parents after this boy went away to college and then we had an opportunity to visit with him when he was in the second year of medical school. He told us, "I'm getting along OK. I still stutter and I still must work every day to keep some blocks from getting away from me. By and large though I have no real problems with it except after I've stayed up all night to study. It's tough then, and some days I don't seem able to do much at all about the blocks, but it's still no real problem. Everbody around here knows I stutter and they accept it even on the bad days. Spelling is still a bit of a problem for me. I have to take extra time to just memorize all the long medical terms. And I'm still a lousy writer. One of the guys up here who was trying to decipher some class notes of mine one time said he bet I could make a fortune tutoring Med students in prescription writing."

## SERVO THEORY

This theory also suggests the possibility of neurological malfunction as the underlying factor in stuttering. It is derived from principles utilized in the development of automatic control systems such as are found in automatic pilot devices, missiles, and computers. It has been hypothesized that the human brain functions in accordance with similar principles for the learning and maintaining of behavior patterns. The general theoretical application of

16 N. Weiner, *The Human Use of Human Beings* (Boston: Houghton Mifflin Co., 1950). What is cybernetics? What is its considered significance for understanding human behavior?

the principles in connection with human behavior has been designated as *information theory.* The more specific im-

17 D. E. Broadbent, *Perception and Communication* (New York: Pergamon Press, 1958). What are the major elements and their functions in information processing?

plications for speech have been termed *servo* or *feedback theory*. Accordingly, as we talk, information is continually

18 Prepare a report on the subject based on a study of G. Fairbanks, "Systematic Research in Experimental Phonetics: 1. A Theory of the Speech Mechanisms as a Servosystem,"*Journal of Speech and Hearing Disorders,* XIX (1954), 133-39; E. D. Mysak, "A Servo Model for Speech Therapy, *Journal of Speech and Hearing Disorders,* XXIV (1959), 144-49; C. Van Riper and J. Irwin, *Voice and Articulation* (Englewood Cliffs, N. J.: Prentice-Hall, Inc., 1958), Chapter 6; R. West, "The Neurophysiology of Speech," in *Handbook of Speech Pathology,* ed. L. E. Travis (New York: Appleton-Century-Crofts, Inc., 1957), Chapter 3.

being fed back to the brain by way of numerous circuits. Some, called *closed circuits* or *cycles,* have all components completely contained within the speaker's organism. They provide the speaker with information about what he just said and how he said it by way of auditory, tactual, and kinesthetic avenues. Others, referred to as *open circuits,* include external components. They (the eyes as well as the ears) check listener reaction. The return flow of information provided by these numerous circuits makes it possible for us to monitor our speech. *Errors* (mispronounced words, too much or too little loudness, incorrect word order, and so forth) normally are caught and corrected automatically. Some such process is presumed essential for any learned behavior system organized in closely connected spatial and temporal units. There just isn't time

19 K. U. Smith, *Delayed Sensory Feedback and Behavior* (Philadelphia, Pa.: W. B. Saunders Co., 1962), pp. 1-15.
What is the *neurogeometric theory* of patterned behavior?

in the normal course of talking for the speaker to pause and check the adequacy of his utterance after each word, or phrase, or even after each sentence. Hence, speech, once learned, becomes self-regulating, with satisfactory monitoring dependent upon the proper functioning and integration of all feedback circuits. Applying the concept to stuttering, Mysak (*23:*188-95) views the disorder as a disturbance of verbalizing-automaticity. He postulates at least four important self-reflexive circuits where disturbances may occur that can be revealed by broken speech.

20 What are these four circuits? How does Mysak utilize the concept to explain other theories of stuttering?

Experimental support for a servo theory of stuttering comes largely from studies of delayed or otherwise distorted auditory feedback. The self-hearing of an utterance, a dimension of feedback called *sidetone*, is the result of receiving sound by way of three separate channels: (*a*) directly through air from the mouth, (*b*) indirectly through air as sound travels out, strikes against reflecting surfaces and back again, and (*c*) through bone and tissue of the head. Now it takes different amounts of time for sound patterns to reach the hearing mechanism by these different routes. This time difference normally is too minute to disturb the integrative process. However, experiments have shown that an imposed delay in sidetone of as much as 0.1 or 0.2 second has profound and dramatic effects on the speech of normal subjects. It can change rate and loudness, distort vocal quality, produce misarticulations, and create fluency disruptions. And, according to Lee (*19:*53-55), the last consist of syllable repetitions like those found among stutterers. Though a later study by Neeley (*24:*63-82) indicated that disruptions which occur in normal speakers and in stutterers under similar conditions of imposed delay are observably different, the possibility remains that stuttering in some instances has its inception in an inherent condition of sidetone delay within the intrinsic circuits.

Stromsta (*30*), for example, has shown that stutterers as a group differ from normal speakers in bone-conduction patterns. There appears to be an interear disparity for stutterers in the phase relationship of bone-tissue sidetone. A similar explanation is suggested by Tomatis (*34:*10-19). His *auricular theory* postulates that neural integration of bilateral auditory feedback normally takes place in the cerebral hemisphere located on the same side as the "directing ear." He claims his research has shown that stuttering is related to a hypoacoustic condition in that ear, thus necessitating a transcerebral transference of auditory neural signals during speaking. The result is a delay in feedback sufficient to disturb integration and create fluency disruptions.

Another study by Stromsta (*31:*286-301), in which he found that distorted sidetone elicited phonatory blockages in normal-speaking subjects, suggests a servo-theory explanation for specific forms of early stuttering. He believes such a condition may explain those cases in which repetitions are characterized by apparent difficulty in initiating or completing the vowel elements and those in which prolongations reveal shifts in the pitch of the vowel being uttered. We have here a possible explanation for the surprising number of cases reported by Bloodstein (*4:*222) in which the earliest signs of stuttering consisted of "hard contacts" and other evidences of literal trouble in uttering words.

Sidetone can also be distorted artificially by acceleration. This causes a speaker to hear his utterances somewhat sooner than is normal. When this happens, speaking rate increases, according to Peters (*26:*483-90). Do we have here a possible explanation for the cluttering symptoms that sometimes precede a problem of stuttering?

In summary, the feedback principle of servo theory offers an interesting new approach to the analysis of learned behavior, both normal and abnormal. The research reviewed by Smith (28) clearly demonstrates the disturbing effects of delayed auditory and visual feedback. Further research doubtless will reveal similar results for other sensory avenues. We can anticipate additional evidence of a relationship between distorted self-hearing and stuttering. We should begin thinking of the implications for prevention and treatment.

### Conflict theory

This theory, developed in detail by Sheehan (*27:* Chapter 3), represents a second major group of ideas about the origin of stuttering that also share a basic premise. They reflect the common belief that stuttering is imposed on essentially normal organisms by intolerable environmental stresses. Sheehan has utilized Miller's (*20:* Chapter 14) four kinds of conflict (approach-approach, avoidance-approach, simple approach-avoidance, and double approach-avoidance) to explain beginning as well as advanced forms of stuttering. The early signs are presumed to represent simple approach-avoidance conflicts. The approach aspect is the need or desire to speak, while the avoidance is a counterpressure involving fear of the consequences. Five separate conflict levels are postulated: word, situation, emotional content, relationship conflict, and ego-protective. Sheehan also believes that guilt feelings have an important role in the onset of stuttering. He states (*27:*135): "Since guilt conspicuously produces blocking in the speech of young children and guilt is an important dynamic in the advanced stutterer, it is likely that guilt feelings lie heavily in the background of the onset of stuttering."

Experimental evidence in support of the approach-avoidance conflict theory has been the source of much valuable knowledge about the confirmed stutterer. Its value beyond a logical theoretical construct for the beginning stutterer requires further research with children. However, the early signs of stuttering in many, many children certainly reveal vacillation and indecision. And we find cases like Michael for whom intimidation creates con-

> Michael at five years of age was reported by the mother to have been showing signs of stuttering for over two years. The father was a policeman who we learned had been transferred from a desk job to the motorcycle unit about the time his son's stuttering began. This seemed an unlikely cause of the trouble until we talked with the father. He was an affable extrovert and it was obvious the boy was the apple of his eye. But we were particularly impressed with his manner of talking. He had a booming voice. We could envision the cowed motorist who heard this policeman say, "Where ya' think you're goin' in such a hurry?" We made a comment about the professional value of his voice and he told us he needed to sound authoritative in his business. "A motorcycle cop has got to scare these law breakers. Otherwise, they just laugh at you or they try to sweet talk you out of a ticket." We couldn't debate that, but wondered if he used the same voice at home. He did, his wife told us, but he was generally so amiable it never occurred to either of them that his manner of talking might sound frightening to their son. However, though neither parent was convinced this could have anything to do with the stuttering, the father was willing to work at monitoring the volume of his voice around the house. We believe it was this single change in his behavior that was responsible for the complete remission of any signs of stuttering in the boy within a period of two months.

flict of one sort or another that generates beginning stuttering behavior.

### STUTTERING AS A NEUROSIS

Conflict also underlies theories reflecting the idea of stuttering as a neurosis. The psychoanalytic concept is exemplary. Psychoanalytic psychiatrists at first stressed the similarity between stuttering and such classic neuroses as hysteria or the various phobias. "More recently, however," Glauber (*13*:93) tells us, "it became generally accepted as a pregenital conversion or a narcissistic neurosis, that is, one in which primarily the executant part of the personality, the ego, is defective or insufficiently developed." The inadequate ego then encounters difficulties in handling demands of the superego. The result is anxiety which, in becoming attached to oral communication because of the close relationship between speech and ego, creates the stuttering. The stuttering symbolizes the conflict. It represents a child's attempts to handle or bind the underlying anxiety.

**21 In the above reference by Glauber, what alternate explanation for stuttering is postulated for some cases? See pp. 96-97.**

Similar explanations, though not couched in orthodox psychoanalytic terminology, are offered by Barbara (*2*) and by Travis (*37:* Chapter 29). Barbara believes the disorder has its seeds in neurotic personalities created by unhealthy family environments. Normal forms and amounts of broken speech are exaggerated because children under such circumstances feel unwanted, unloved, weak, insecure, and inadequate. According to Travis (*37*:919), "Stuttering may be defined as an advertisement of strong, unconscious motives of which the stutterer is deeply ashamed." The stutterer, he believes, is the individual who as a very young child simply couldn't cope with the socializing demands of his culture. It was too harsh and hostile. The result was repression of his true feelings. The stuttering then emerges because he is fearful of revealing the awful thoughts he harbors about himself and other members of his family.

### THE SELF-PROCESS THEORY

A closely related concept of stuttering is presented by Murphy and Fitzsimons (22). They, too, claim the early stuttering behavior arises from anxiety. Impaired interpersonal relationships are presumed to be the source of conflict that creates the anxiety. However, though stut-

22 What do Murphy and Fitzsimons mean by the self-process? What can you find about the self-concept for comparison? Your best bet is a text on child growth and development. For a start, you might try B. R. McCandless, *Children and Adolescents* (New York: Holt, Rinehart and Winston, Inc., 1961), Chapter 6.

For another explanation of stuttering with an interpersonal relationship basis, see G. Wyatt, "Stammering and Language Learning in Early Childhood," *Journal of Abnormal and Social Psychology,* XLIV (1949), 75-84.

terers are considered to be generally somewhat below average in their early emotional adjustments, these writers do not believe the neurotic label is justified.

Stuttering to Murphy and Fitzsimons (22:145) ". . . is a learned, nonintegrative, self-defensive reaction to anxiety or fear of threatening circumstances with which the person feels incapable of coping." Five general sources of the underlying anxiety are suggested: (*a*) suppression or domination sufficient to threaten self-autonomy, (*b*) extreme and chronic inconsistency of adult handling, (*c*) too many experiences characterized by derogation, belittling, or rejection, (*d*) complete lack of external controls, and (*e*) fears and guilt feelings generated by a child's reactions to the foregoing experiences. Specific causes are thought to be multiple and complex, ". . . lying in a diffuse constellation of dynamic forces which revolve around basic life processes and the degree of success with which a given child meets the challenges of speech and related developmental tasks" (*22:*154).

The result is a child who is confused and chronically concerned about adult evaluations of his behavior. The anxiety initially need not be directly associated with speech per se. It can be related to most any developing skill or self-image. Thus, beginning stuttering in some instances may reflect anxiety about such various things as appearance, muscular strength, or language skills. Pronounced apprehension about any felt inadequacy can cause a child to be generally hesitant in his behavior. And when he speaks, the hesitancy may be manifested in broken fluency. This doubtless is the explanation for many cases of early stuttering in which the behavior disappears before developing into serious communication problems. As adequate skills and satisfactory self-images are acquired, the hesitancy disappears. Also, this may explain why stuttering sometimes begins or reappears in the early adolescent years. This is a time when most children are troubled by a host of adjustment problems which they feel must be solved in a short time and without the help of parents whenever possible.

In summary, here again we have a group of theories supported by the logic of their fundamental constructs, but so far unable to be validated by experimental research as the explanation for beginning stuttering in all or even the majority of cases. However, here also too many cases are encountered that illustrate the general tenets of these theories too clearly for us to deny their validity as a source of stuttering—cases like Marsha.

Marsha, a highly intelligent nine-year-old only child, had been stuttering severely for over four years. The father had deserted the family the year Marsha was born. The mother had gone to work in the small variety store owned by her father and had taken over its management two years later when he died. She worked long hours and usually did the bookkeeping on Sundays. Marsha was cared for by her grandmother, a sour, sharp-tongued woman plagued by painful arthritis. She complained constantly about the way her daughter ran the store and about being tied down to housework and the care of a child who she frequently claimed never should have been born. She seldom allowed Marsha to have other children in the house. When others called to invite Marsha to their homes, the grandmother would be agreeable, but then would warn the caller that Marsha would have to be watched closely because she didn't know how to behave yet.

We viewed this situation as a "parent trap" problem. The mother was economically bound to the store and emotionally as well as economically bound to the home situation. She couldn't leave either place. We assuaged her guilt feelings as best as we could and she agreed to see if she could find a high-school or college student who could work on Fridays from four to nine o'clock, leaving her some special time each week to devote exclusively to her daughter. We then worked directly with Marsha for about two months and succeeded in helping her learn to control the worst of the grimaces that contorted her face when she stuttered. She also became less embarrassed about the stuttering. That was all we felt could be accomplished with this case at the time. We hoped Marsha could return or have an opportunity for treatment elsewhere when she was older and could be helped with the underlying emotional problems.

### Evaluational theory

This theory, known also as the *semantic* or *diagnostic theory*, reflects a belief in the essential constitutional and psychological normalcy of stutterers. It also emphasizes the idea that stuttering is imposed upon children who in nearly every instance have perfectly normal speech. A fundamental premise of this theory is that normal forms and amounts of broken speech are recognized erroneously by associates of some children as abnormal and undesirable. Stuttering then actually has its source in the resulting mal-attitudes and penalizing reactions of a child's close associates, usually, of course, his parents. It is considered similar to iatrogenic, or "physician induced," illnesses in the medical field. According to Johnson (*14*:246), stuttering with but few exceptions literally doesn't exist until after it has been diagnosed.

The concept has been the target of a great deal of research that has contributed invaluable knowledge about stuttering. One extensive collection of studies has indicated that stuttering generally is found only in societies that reveal a notable lack of tolerance for fluency disruptions in children. Indeed, some societies have no equivalent

23 W. Johnson, "The Indians Have No Word for it: Stuttering in Children," *Quarterly Journal of Speech,* XXX (1944), 330-37.

A. K. Bullen, "A Cross Cultural Approach to the Problem of Stuttering," *Child Development,* XVI (1945), 1-88.

J. C. Snidicor, "Why the Indian Does Not Stutter," *Quarterly Journal of Speech,* XXXIII (1947), 493-95.

E. M. Lemert, "Some Indians Who Stutter," *Journal of Speech and Hearing Disorders,* XVIII (1953), 168-74.

J. J. Morgenstern, "Socio-economic Factors in Stuttering," *Journal of Speech and Hearing Disorders,* XXI (1956), 25-33.

J. L. Stewart, "The Problem of Stuttering in Certain North American Indian Societies," *Journal of Speech and Hearing Disorders,* Monograph Supplement No. 6 (April 1960), pp. 1-66.

What specific contributions to evaluational theory are provided by each of these studies? What other supportive evidence can you find?

word for stuttering or stammering in their language. Repetitive utterances in young children are not merely tolerated. In some instances they actually are encouraged. Few people with the problem of fluency we call *stuttering* are to be found in these societies.

Additional support for the theory comes from another group of studies of parent attitudes in our own culture. Significant discrepancies were revealed in the standards for acceptable developmental behavior including the fluency of speech. Most parents, unless they have had personal

24 For detailed accounts of relevant research, see W. Johnson and R. Leutenegger, eds., *Stuttering in Children and Adults: Thirty Years of Research at the University of Iowa* (Minneapolis: University of Minnesota Press, 1955), and W. Johnson, *The Onset of Stuttering* (Minneapolis: University of Minnesota Press), 1959.

Compare the case for evaluational theory with M. E. Wingate, "Evaluation and Stuttering, Part I: Speech Characteristics of Young Children," *Journal of Speech and Hearing Disorders,* XXVII (1962), 106-15, and "Part II: Environmental Stress and Critical Appraisal of Speech," *Journal of Speech and Hearing Disorders,* XXVII (1962), 244-57.

acquaintance with stuttering, disregard the broken speech that occurs when their children talk. They do not question its normalcy. The few who do are inclined to be perfectionistic and dominating. The latter trait, Moncur (*21:* 155-65) believes, includes "domination by disciplinary action, domination by oversupervising and overprotecting the child, domination by holding the child to excessively high standards, and domination by adverse parental criticism."

Evaluational theory has been widely accepted in this country. In fact, it is one of two basic points of view concerning the significance of repetitions and other early forms of broken speech in relation to stuttering. Evaluation theorists claim stuttering usually is created by listeners who mistake normal fluency disruptions for beginning signs of stuttering. Representatives of the other viewpoint, while not denying the evil effects of such labels as stuttering or stammering on those to whom the term is applied, believe parents frequently are justified in the initial concern about their children's speech. They believe there is sufficient evidence to indicate that the broken speech in many instances is noticeably different from that of most children. It is considered to be excessive in amount and/or

25 See R. West, "An Agnostic's Speculations about Stuttering," in *Stuttering: A Symposium,* ed. J. Eisenson (New York: Harper & Row, Publishers, 1958), pp. 193-96; O. Bloodstein, "The Development of Stuttering: I, Changes in Nine Basic Features," *Journal of Speech and Hearing Disorders,* XXV (1960), 221; C. Van Riper, *Speech Correction, Principles and Methods,* 4th ed. (Englewood Cliffs, N. J.: Prentice-Hall, Inc., 1963), p. 328; C. Bluemel, *The Riddle of Stuttering* (Danville, Ill.: Interstate Publishing Co., 1957), p. 31; M. E. Wingate, "Evaluation and Stuttering, Part I: Speech Characteristics of Young Children," *Journal of Speech and Hearing Disorders,* XXVII (1962), 106-15.

frequency and also may differ in form. Repetitions in these children are more likely to occur on syllables and sounds while those of other children typically are of whole words and phrases.

The observed differences between early and later forms of stuttering lead advocates of this school of thought to adopt Bluemel's (5:91-102) concept of stuttering as a disorder of two distinct stages which he termed *primary* and *secondary. Primary stutterers* became the designation for those cases, almost always young children, with relatively mild though excessive or frequent repetitions and prolongations who were thought to be unaware and unconcerned about the broken speech. *Secondary stutterers* then were those individuals with more noticeable forms of the disorder that developed after they began to react emotionally to breaks in the fluency of their speech. Evalua-

26 A third stage was introduced in 1954. What was it? What was its significance? See C. Van Riper, *Speech Correction, Principles and Methods,* 3rd ed. (Englewood Cliffs, N. J.: Prentice-Hall, Inc., 1954), pp. 365-69.

**Has there been any change in that writer's ideas about stages of stuttering? If so, what? See C. Van Riper, *Speech Correction, Principles and Methods,* 4th ed. (Englewood Cliffs, N. J.: Prentice-Hall, Inc., 1963), pp. 327-48.**

tion theorists tend to deny the validity of this dichotomous classification. Their conception of stuttering doesn't include the primary stage. Speaker awareness colored by distress is assumed before the label of stutterer or stammerer is applicable. As Johnson states (*14*:216), "Stuttering is an anticipatory, apprehensive, hypertonic avoidance reaction."

This controversy, as we mentioned earlier, remains unresolved. We believe both concepts are right, though neither is applicable for as many cases as the more ardent advocates of the theories claim. Some children have histories of stuttering, i.e., they have periodically exhibited frequent or excessive amounts of broken speech, without evidence that anyone has reacted to it as anything but normal. And stuttering develops in some individuals in spite of ideal environments and the most skillful professional help. On the other hand, a regrettable number of children are encountered who are in grave danger of becoming stutterers because some adult is creating unjustified concern about broken speech that falls well within normal limits. Some do not escape. Sometimes the unfortunate labeling is done by a parent, as illustrated by Van Riper (*38*:320):

> We first met the child at the age of three. He was brought to us by his mother, a former college speech teacher. She was tense and anxious about the boy, claiming that he was beginning to stutter. In three hours of observation, play and parent conversation, we were unable to find anything but an occasional repetition of a phrase or whole word, usually under conditions of word choice which would have made

any adult hesitate. Each time one of these occurred, she would roll her eyes or tug at our sleeve to point out the stuttering. Knowing that stuttering is intermittent, we even introduced some experimental stress, hurrying the child, interrupting, rejecting his statements, and averting our attention.

Recognizing the mother's anxiety, and being as careful as possible, we tried to reassure and educate her concerning the prevalence of repetition and hesitation in most children's speech. We made available some parental counseling to help her face her own problems, but she refused to participate. Said she, "You're just like everyone else. Every doctor and speech therapist I've taken Ricky to has said the same thing. You can't fool a child's own mother. He's stuttering and you know it."

A year later she brought the child back to the clinic, and sure enough, he was stuttering with all the abnormality of an adult. "See!" she said triumphantly, "I told you he was a stutterer all the time."

Sometimes the culprit is a classroom teacher:

The mother of a second grader once came to us concerned because her daughter, who had never shown any previous signs, was beginning to stutter. She and her husband hadn't been paying any attention to it until the teacher, in a recent conference, had commented about the girl's stuttering and had asked if anything was being done about it. The mother said the teacher told her she had noticed a little trouble early in the year and immediately had begun to stop her whenever any occurred and asked her to start over and to talk more slowly. As the girl began to have more trouble in the classroom, the teacher reported she had had a friendly talk with Dianne about what a serious problem stuttering was and encouraged her to try harder to keep from having that kind of trouble when she talked.

And sometimes, improbable as it should be, it is a speech therapist who is responsible for creating stuttering.

27 See W. Johnson, "Language and Speech Hygiene," *General Semantics Monograph*, I (Chicago: Institute of General Semantics, 1939), p. 38. Also W. Johnson, "Letter to the Editor," Journal of Speech *and Hearing Disorders*, XIV (1949), 175.

## SUMMARY

We believe the available experimental and clinical evidence indicates that stuttering has its origin in a variety of conditions and/or circumstances. It may reflect the effects of some fundamental and irreversible biologic difference. It may be caused by an immaturity of certain organic systems or personality components that prevents the acquisition of normal forms of speech or language at the expected age levels. It may have its source in a child's emotional reactions to a developmental problem such as delayed speech or faulty articulation. Or it may be imposed on a normal organism and normal behavior by intolerable environmental stresses.

The gradual onset, the intermittency, and the similarity of beginning signs of stuttering among children create grave problems for research and for clinical diagnosis. Until more is known about the origin of this disorder, therapists' decisions about etiology must rest on evidence obtained from careful investigation of each case.

### SIGNIFICANCE OF CHANGE

WHATEVER MAY BE ITS SOURCE, STUTTERING SELDOM REMAINS static. It grows. And as it grows, it tends to change in form as well as in severity. Early patterns are replaced, obscured, or supplemented by more pronounced and abnormal behavior. Repetitions or prolongations become troublesome "blocks." Tremors may appear in certain oral structures. Word attempts may be interrupted and replaced with synonyms. Reattempts on words may be prefaced by noticeable pauses during which a child can appear to be experiencing some sort of silent internal struggle. Some children become less talkative and occasionally may refuse to speak.

# 3 *advanced stuttering*

Such changes signal the onset of the advanced stage of this disorder. They reveal much about the nature of stuttering and its impact on the speaker and the listener. Beginning stuttering seldom disrupts communication enough to justify being considered anything more than a minor behavioral difference, but advanced patterns of stuttering more often than not mean that the difficulty is on its way to becoming a genuine clinical problem. It is the overt and covert behavior associated with the advanced stage that constitute the social as well as the literal communication-handicapped portions of this disorder in nearly all cases. When stuttering can be restricted to the disruptions that characterize the early stage, direct clinical treatment seldom is required. In fact, it is not uncommon for the signs of early stuttering to disappear spontaneously. But when advanced patterns appear and particularly when they have become firmly established, the chances of remission are slight without expert professional attention.

Though marked controversy still exists about the origin of beginning stuttering, there is general agreement among speech pathologists that advanced patterns are learned. They are reflections of a more or less conscious and desperate attempt to solve a problem. The fact that they generally serve to create more complicated and distressing problems indicates their critical importance to the disorder. Understanding why and how these new patterns are acquired is essential for effective treatment of stutterers.

### ORIGINS OF CHANGES: CONCERN AND FRUSTRATION

The advanced forms of stuttering are initiated when early patterns of broken speech become objects of concern or frustration to the speaker. *Concern is here defined as an adverse feeling associated with anticipation of an unpleasant experience; frustration is a similar feeling but related to an unpleasant experience presently occurring.* Feelings of concern are engendered by experiences associated with actual or imagined penalties. They are then later precipitated by thoughts of similar reactions in subsequent situations. Feelings of frustration occur as some obstacle or obstruction is encountered during the actual pursuit of a goal. They are experienced when we are seeking to accomplish something and find ourselves blocked from satisfactory completion of the activity. Either of these emotional reactions may be experienced over a wide range of degrees. Mild concern usually is experienced as a vague feeling of uneasiness, greater amounts as nervous apprehension, while acute feelings of concern are likely to be experienced as fear or even panic. Slight amounts of frustration create relatively mild feelings of annoyance or irritation. Greater amounts tend to evoke anger, or rage, and hostility.

The emotions of concern or frustration become interrelated in time like chickens and eggs. Each may beget the other. Anger, for example, is known to be a common mask for fear or anxiety, as Sullivan (*33*:135) has shown. Likewise, concern can generate feelings of frustration. Guilt feelings then may add potent ingredients to the explosive mixture. We need to understand all we can about these feelings, how they may be evoked, how they serve to precipitate behavior changes, and how those changes affect the stutterer as well as his stuttering.

### The significance of concern and frustration

Signs of concern or frustration may signify many things, all of them threatening. Any threat to life or limb understandably produces emotional amalgamations of pronounced fear and anger. So does the threat of losing one's means of financial support. Lives and incomes are essential possessions and risk of losing either can be emotionally disastrous. Fortunately, such threats are relatively infrequent occurrences, but they do happen. However, there is

A severe stutterer once told us this story: "I stuttered some until I was in high school. Then I got some valuable help, and I thought it was gone for good. I seldom had any trouble at all for several years. I was working as a fireman on a locomotive in a switch yard. One day we were using a stretch of the main line to switch some cars. We didn't know of any train due on that line for another half hour. I looked out to check something and suddenly saw a freight bearing right down on us. My engineer was busy inside the cab.

I tried to tell him, but I couldn't say a word. I couldn't even stutter before it was too late. The freight wasn't going very fast, but both locomotives were wrecked. Nobody was killed, but my partner lost a leg. I've never forgiven myself. If only I could have warned him." This man was still stuttering severely eight years later when we knew him. We were unable to help and neither was a psychiatrist to whom we referred this case.

another highly prized possession that for many is a daily source of emotional upset. We refer to self-esteem, that critically important ingredient of self-confidence, morale, and mental health. Self-esteem is the barometer of interpersonal relationships. Each person's regard for himself reflects what he sees in the mirrors of other people's eyes. Toleration by others is seldom enough. To build self-esteem we must have acceptance at least, approbation or accolade at best. The required acceptance tends to depend on satisfactory answers to three questions: Are physical endowments normal enough? Is control over one's organism adequate for desired behavior? Is behavior within the perceived norms? Unsatisfactory answers to one or more of these questions can create troublesome amounts of concern or frustration. Too much deviation in appearance, self control, and/or behavior threaten self-esteem. We have

28 About being different and its consequences, Wendell Johnson tells us, "A difference to be a difference has to make a difference." We have worked effectively with some adult stutterers by providing little more than the suggestion that they find out more about this cryptically profound statement by reading his book, *People in Quandaries* (New York: Harper & Row, Publishers, Inc., 1946). We suggest you read it, too, particularly Chapters 1, 2, 5, and 11.

known individuals with cleft lips and palates who considered their facial disfigurements far greater tragedies than the speech defects associated with them. We have worked with cerebral palsied cases for whom the agonizing frustration of trying to control unruly muscles became so unbearable they gave up. And regarding the importance of behavior being within the perceived norms, every speech therapist knows his job has been accomplished when his case becomes convinced that people no longer notice anything wrong when he talks. The difference that once made a difference no longer does so. He can now enjoy the pleasures of acceptance, satisfying interpersonal relationships, and more adequate feelings of self-esteem.

## SOURCES OF CONCERN ABOUT BROKEN SPEECH

### *1. Verbal Labels*

Feelings of concern about fluency disruptions are created in many children by adverse listener reactions. These reactions can be verbal or nonverbal in form. Among the most harmful verbal reactions is the attaching of the label *stuttering* to the broken speech of a young child. The words of any language have the meanings people give them. In our society, many individuals associate stuttering, at least in its more obvious or bizarre forms, with ridicule, rejection, and pity. They think of Porky the Pig, who is considered funny because he stutters. They recall actors like Roscoe Ates who stuttered to provide comic relief in movies. Or they may remember published accounts about people's lives that emphasized frustration, embarrassment, and social penalty experienced as a result of stuttering. Parents understandably want their children to be spared from such misery. However, many fail to understand that the meaning they attribute to a word is conveyed to their children when the word is used. Thus, when early fluency disruptions are labeled as *stuttering*, the word can eventually evoke the same concern in the child that it signifies for the parent.

An interesting indication of differences in words with similar meanings may be noted in some parents and stutterers who prefer the word *stammering* for difficulties of fluency. This term generally doesn't suggest the same penalty-evoking behavior as stuttering. Some believe stam-

29 In another volume of this series, *Cluttering* by Deso Weiss, the author refuses to use the word *stuttering* and insists on the word *stammering*. Why?

mering refers to a distinctly different disorder; others associate it with breaks in speech but not in forms or amounts that disturb the listener. We once worked with a college student who insisted during the initial interview that his problem was a stammer that bothered him at times. He did not have a great deal of difficulty, but he did show some of the covert behavior of the confirmed stutterer and on occasion would exhibit mild lip tremors at the beginnings of words. We talked for a time and finally decided to ask if he had ever thought of his difficulty as stuttering. He immediately began to have more trouble as he denied the validity of that label for him. He told us he had known people who stuttered and he was certain he never had "that kind of a problem." His concern about being a stutterer was obvious and we didn't press the point. However, in subsequent treatment sessions, he admitted knowing he stuttered, but he said it was much easier to bear as long as he could call it stammering. He told us he had refused on two occasions to go to a summer camp for stutterers because he didn't want to have to associate with others who had that problem.

Similar accounts reflecting the adverse influence of that particular label are encountered frequently among older stutterers. Some avoid any label by telling people they just have trouble saying some words or by simply stating they don't know what their problem is. Few people with established stuttering problems can react unemotionally to the words *stutter* and *stuttering*. Most harbor intense hatred for these words; for some, the feelings about "being a stutterer" become the dominant feature of the clinical problem. These feelings may be acquired early in the course of this disorder and, as we pointed out earlier, there is little doubt that the attachment of an evil label to broken speech is capable of creating sufficient concern to generate stuttering.

### *2. Other Verbal Evaluations*

The literal use of specific labels isn't necessary. There are many other ways to tell a child he is doing something he shouldn't, when he talks, that can be equally harmful. Well meaning parents who know about the dangers of labeling and conscientiously work to avoid having speech referred to as stuttering or stammering may unknowingly create concern by responding to the occurrence of broken speech with such comments as, "Now, let's try not to go so fast when we talk" or "If you'll just go a little slower, all those words will come out more smoothly." The long

**30** **What other verbal reactions have been reported by parents of stutterers? See W. Johnson, *The Onset of Stuttering* (Minneapolis: University of Minnesota Press, 1959), Appendixes, pp. 87-90.**

ears of children can overhear conversation when parents believe they are fast asleep. One stutterer told us, "I remember very vividly when I first felt there was something wrong. I was in bed and heard my mother telling my father about the trouble I had trying to tell her about something that happened at school that day. She said I had an awful time and that it almost made her cry. I heard them talk about a speech therapist and whether they should take me to see one. I don't recall having to go to one at that time so they must have changed their minds or else I got better, but I sure remember laying there in bed that night wondering what was wrong and what was going to happen to me."

Thus, labels and other comments that imply abnormality or carry other threats of social penalty can be harmful. However, it isn't always the actual words that do the damage. The manner in which they are said may be the alarm bell. Voices communicate emotions. They often tell a child more than words. "Now, Henry," for example, has several meanings, depending on the way the speaker sounds. It can mean, "I want you to do that immediately—*right now.*" It can signify, "You really don't expect me to believe that, do you?" or, "Let's be a good boy and share our toys." It also can mean, "How many times must I remind you to slow down when you're talking?"

But we must not be too quick to blame parents for children's stuttering. Comments that convince a child there is something wrong with his speech can come from other people. They may come from playmates who happen to select a siege of excessive fumbling, hesitancy, or repeating as the target of teasing when their friend has become a momentary enemy or victim. At times a child's innocent statement, "You talk funny," can create the beginnings of concern that lead to a more serious problem. Also, brothers or sisters may find unusual amounts of broken speech to be a handy subject for fanning flames of sibling rivalry and competition for parental attention.

### *3. Nonverbal Reactions*

There are numerous forms of nonverbal behavior which can be equally effective in creating concern about broken speech. A scowl, a look of despair or of undue solicitude as a child's speech is disrupted by hesitancies or repetitions may focus emotion-laden attention on the fragmented behavior. Sometimes nonverbal reactions are purposely contrived and consciously applied by parents or other associates in well meant attempts to prevent children from becoming highly aware of disfluent speech or the listener's concern. Unfortunately, some people do not sufficiently appreciate the perceptiveness or sensitivity of some youngsters. The fawn knows instantly when the doe freezes.

Others, because of their own concern and eagerness to prevent the development of a serious problem, overdo reactions which might well be effective in more moderate amounts. Speech therapists frequently encounter classroom teachers who believe they are helping young stutterers not only by never mentioning the difficulty in the children's presence, but also by never calling on them for participation in recitations or discussions. Such complete separation from one's classmates can be puzzling if not downright distressing to some children. And if these children conclude they are being avoided because of the way they talk at times, the broken speech can quickly become an object of concern.

31 For additional implications of this reaction see C. Van Riper, *Speech Correction, Principles and Methods*, 4th ed. (Englewood Cliffs, N. J.: Prentice-Hall, Inc., 1963), p. 377.

A striking example of an exaggerated response to early stuttering was provided by the mother of a four-year-old girl with whom we once worked. This parent had a slight stuttering problem herself and was well aware of the possible dangers of labels and critical comments. She felt she always was very careful about reacting to her daughter's speech in any way that could contribute to concern about it. During the initial visit to our clinic, the mother and child were observed through a two-way mirror as they became acquainted with available toys. Interaction was free and easy. This mother played easily and unselfconsciously with her daughter even in the presence of known but unseen observers. However, we noted that whenever the child stumbled or repeated, the mother abruptly became silent and waited until the girl was talking smoothly again. Occasionally she even stopped in the middle of one of her own sentences. Sometimes the girl would then stop too and seem to be waiting for a sentence to be completed, but the mother always remained calmly silent until the child had gone on and was talking fluently.

In subsequent discussions with the mother, we asked how she usually reacted to the occurrence of any stuttering in her daughter. She told us: "Well, I never say anything about it. I know that can be bad. I try to make her feel that she has all the time in the world to speak and to give her my full attention." We agreed with the wisdom of these responses and sensed that she was unaware of overdoing her reactions. Also, we assumed it was possible this parent harbored some guilt feelings about having a child with a problem like her own, so we said nothing more about the matter until several weeks later when we felt she was ready to be confronted with a taped recording of the play activity. She was able to listen objectively by that time and finally interrupted the recording to say:

"Heavens! Do I do that all the time? I wouldn't have believed anybody who told me I was being so obvious by being silent so long or so often. I have noticed that Mary sometimes seems to stutter more when I've stopped and am waiting for her to get through some trouble, but I never imagined it had anything to do with my silence." With this parent it turned out to be easy to discuss less obvious ways of applying the two commendable ideas of providing attention and time. However, even with the mother's changed behavior, this child's stuttering persisted and it became necessary to apply direct treatment methods when she entered school. There were other factors in this case (there nearly always are!), including possibly an inherited predisposition for stuttering, but we believe the frequent exaggerated silences of the mother contributed considerably to the development of an established problem in this girl.

The self-unawareness of behavior evident in this parent is not uncommon. Such responses often occur unconsciously, particularly when verbal responses are being consciously inhibited. In such circumstances, thoughts and attitudes can be vividly conveyed by silent "ayes" and "nays." Every individual tends to have a characteristic nonverbal mannerism that serves to release tension when he is trying to avoid revealing his feelings. It may be a blinking or shifting of eyes, a movement of hand or arm, a general postural shift, or a slight but perceptible change in facial expression. Fortune tellers have known this for centuries and have used the knowledge to amaze people with information obtained by the simple device of making numerous general statements and watching for the silent reactions that let them know which items apply. Experienced interviewers utilize similar observational skills to help them refrain from exploring sensitive areas too quickly. Speech therapists also must be alert to nonverbal reactions of concern that may be contributing to some child's development of a stuttering problem and must become skillful in identifying them for the people involved.

### Self-generated feelings of concern

It is not always possible to find valid evidence of penalizing listener reactions to explain the obvious concern some children reveal about early difficulties in talking. However skillful and intensive the search may be, sometimes no evidence either within or outside the family can be found to support that common explanation for the emotional reactions. Some other source of concern is indicated in these cases. We believe the harmful awareness for these children first began when they were learning to talk or struggling to establish adequate relationships. Fractured fluency may begin very early.

Parents of young stutterers sometimes (surprisingly frequently, in fact) report the presence of greater amounts of sensitivity in these children. We are not surprised, of course, to hear about shyness and other signs of sensitiveness after stuttering has become something of a social problem to a child, but these parents frequently report that their youngsters were noticeably more sensitive from early infancy. Case histories for these children commonly include the information that they have always cried more easily and more often than others in the family, that they were quickly and easily frustrated, and that their feelings were easily hurt. They are often described as children who "had to be handled with kid gloves," who seemed to need undue amounts of affection and attention. In short, they have been what are commonly called *sensitive* children.

Sensitivity is not easy to define and we cannot explain

why some children seem almost to be born with too much of whatever it is, though often we discover close relatives who are much the same way. We offer an operational, or

32 What is said about this by P. J. Glasner, "Personality Characteristics and Emotional Problems in Stutterers under the Age of Five," *Journal of Speech and Hearing Disorders,* XIV (1949), 135-38? Compare with R. West, "An Agnostic's Speculations about Stuttering," in *Stuttering: A Symposium,* ed. J. Eisenson (New York: Harper & Row, Publishers, Inc., 1958), pp. 185-90.

working, definition. Thus, *sensitivity* in its developed forms, is here defined as a *hyperalertness to the adequacy of one's behavior coupled with something less than normal ability to tolerate unfavorable reactions by others.* Sensitive people more or less desperately want to avoid critical evaluations. They continually seek open and obvious signs of approval, and reactions that aren't patently favorable may be interpreted as criticism. And they tend to be constantly scanning their own behavior for signs of anything unusual, anything that possibly might evoke undesirable reactions.

33 A possibility exists that this sensitivity may originate in the nonverbal communication experiences prior to the onset of speech. See the booklet *Stuttering: Its Prevention* by the Speech Foundation of America (8:13).

Such a trait, if it may be called that, potentially has a dual role in the evolution of established stuttering problems. First, by causing a child very early in his life to be more unsure, more cautious, more hesitant, sensitivity may sometimes underly the anxiety mentioned earlier as a source of beginning stuttering. It later also becomes the source of advanced forms of the disorder because of his pressing need to avoid any questionable behavior. The sensitive child is more likely to be highly conscious of the way he talks just as he is more highly aware and evaluative of other behavior. And if a day happens to come along during which he hears excessive amounts of breaks in his speech, and particularly if it is during a period of special alertness, genuine concern may become focused on the fluency disruptions. No adverse listener reactions to speech may be needed. The concern in a very literal sense may be self-generated.

### Fractured fluency as a source of frustration

Advanced stuttering may develop in some children who have never sensed the concern of others about speech. Some children (and occasionally adults) reveal obvious signs of advanced stuttering yet show little or no evidence of concern about their difficulties. The stuttering of these people may include eye blinks, head jerks, gasping, or other complicated overt symptoms, but patterns for the majority will be characterized by pronounced tension-postures and struggle behavior in the oral area. The stuttering tends to occur frequently and sometimes is quite severe, yet these cases may talk freely if not smoothly. They do not seem highly concerned about being stutterers, about having something wrong with their speech that is socially undesirable. Instead, if anything, they feel frustrated in their efforts to talk smoothly. Bloodstein (*4*:222) tells of encountering children as young as age two or three who already showed signs of advanced stuttering for which concern could not be the logical source. The information suggests that some children perceive early fluency disruptions as literal impediments. If so, reactions of frustration would be the natural consequence.

34 Compare with W. Johnson, *The Onset of Stuttering* (Minneapolis: University of Minnesota Press, 1959), p. 258.

Most of us have known how aggravating it can be to find ourselves even momentarily blocked from satisfactorily completing some important or pleasant activity. Typewriter keys stick. The ball point pen won't write. Frustration can be an exceedingly annoying experience and its sequelae often serve only to add more distress. The frustrated adult tends to be an angry one. Aggression unleashes the beast in all of us. We attack others or ourselves. We also become more tense, less able to think clearly, and we become less efficient and skillful.

The frustrated child also reacts with anger and aggressive behavior. He, too, is likely to strike back with forceful vigor at the perceived source of his frustration. A three-year-old, unsuccessful in making a tower of alphabet blocks, may suddenly whack the whole pile into all corners. Or one too many failures to draw a suitable picture of the family pet can result in a whole pan full of mutilated crayons.

Angry hostility vented on uncooperative crayons can resolve that particular frustration, at least until the destruction is discovered by an anguished mother who may quickly prove how universal it is to battle directly with the people or the things that create feelings of frustration. But

35 The student of stuttering needs to acquire special understanding of frustration. Its effects will be encountered in one or more of its numerous guises in clinical work with nearly every case. Basic information on various theories and the relevant research is available in K. Lewin, *A Dynamic Theory of Personality* (New York: McGraw-Hill Book Company, Inc., 1935); J. Dollard et. al., *Frustration and Aggression* (London: Kegan, Paul, Trench, Trubner and Co., Ltd., 1944); N. R. F. Maier, *Frustration: The Study of Behavior Without a Goal* (New York: McGraw-Hill Book Company, Inc., 1949).

Reviews and critiques of the work on frustration may be found in B. McCandless, *Children and Adolescents* (New York: Holt, Rinehart and Winston, Inc., 1961); A. J. Yates, *Frustration and Conflict* (London: Methuen and Co., Ltd., 1962); volumes of *The Annual Review of Psychology*.

the child who tries to overcome frustrating disruptions in fluency by forcefully attacking the unmanageable words is in for more trouble immediately. As he struggles with increasing tension in lips, tongue, or larynx, he finds talking more and more difficult. Van Riper (*38*:330) presents a vivid and detailed picture of the manner in which reactions to frustration engendered by early experiences with broken speech may generate greater difficulty. He believes the resulting struggle leads to actual tremors in musculatures of the articulatory structures. The tremors cause a child to feel literally blocked in his efforts to talk. Feelings of frustration change to fear. Fear may change to panic. Escape is sought in any possible way. Unfortunately, the very devices that release the tremor and free the child to talk serve only to complicate his problem.

36 The whole idea of tremors as a significant factor in the development of stuttering should challenge the research-minded student. It is not unduly difficult for most normal-speaking adults to induce tremors in their own articulatory mechanisms and momentarily experience what seems to be happening in some stuttering. Try this: get set for the initial sound of some word that begins with *t*. Then, just as you prepare to initiate the movements associated with starting the word, jam your tongue against that surface of your mouth with which it is in contact. Keep pushing forcefully as you simultaneously try to start the word. Deadlock? Impasse? Tremors?

Try the same thing on a word or two that begins with *p*, *b*, or *d*. On some word attempt did you suddenly find your mouth locked in a tremor that for a time was out of control? If this is what happens to stutterers, is not frustration, fear, or even panic an understandable reaction? But are they the same things? Are the "tiny little vibrations" Van Riper mentions miniature forms of these simulated tremors or of the genuine ones easily observed in some stutterers? If so, by what means can their existence in young children be objectively verified?

Van Riper may be right, but we believe an alternate course may be followed by some cases. Bloodstein's (*4*:221) account of stuttering development indicates a relatively common tendency for prolongations as well as for complete stoppages to be present in conjunction with repetitive patterns which presumably have been present for some time. Though we must keep in mind that Bloodstein's was a cross-sectional rather than a longitudinal study of early stuttering, his observations still suggest the possibility that reactions of some children to repetitive patterns result in prolonged word elements rather than in tremors.

37 Or do we possibly have here a difference in reactions to tremors determined by the type of sound involved? If not, what is the significance of comments by Bloodstein (*4*:222) about the kinds of sounds prominently involved in hard contacts (of which he considers prolongations one aspect) and by Van Riper (*38*:330) about the sounds associated with early signs of tremors?

## Effects of concern and frustration

When listener penalties, adverse self-evaluations, or communication impairment are sufficient to be threatening and thus to evoke emotional reactions of concern or frustration about fluency disruptions, the result is more or less frantic effort to avoid the noxious behavior. "More or less" has considerable significance here because neither concern nor frustration, per se, leads necessarily to changes that result in troublesome stuttering problems. Some children are encountered who have been stuttering for some time and show signs of an advanced stage yet are not sufficiently bothered by the difficulty to be motivated to do anything about it. Similar cases are found occasionally among adults who have stuttered for many years. These people usually will verbalize some feelings of concern about the difficulty, and some will admit they would prefer not to stutter (others will say they would prefer not to be stutterers!), but their attitudes indicate quite clearly that the stuttering has not been any real problem to them.

The point is that emotional feelings about broken speech are not always harmful. Mild amounts may affect both the frequency and the form of stuttering, yet not result in problems that justify clinical treatment. In fact, great harm may be done by treating these people, and we shall have more to say later about the importance of caution in assuming that the obvious presence of stuttering along with concern about it signifies a problem.

38 Meanwhile, we suggest you learn more about the distinction between stuttering as a *defect* and as a *problem* by reading J. J. Villarreal, "Two Aspects of Stuttering Therapy," *Journal of Speech and Hearing Disorders*, XV (1950), pp. 215-20.

### The spiral effect

Pronounced feelings of concern or frustration are another matter. They generate greater amounts of broken speech. Repetitions become more numerous. Prolongations are extended. Hesitancy contributes its own additional element of disfluency. The increased amount of broken speech intensifies adverse listener reactions and self-awareness. The breaks in speech are now vividly sensed. They begin to ring in the ears. The emotional reactions now associated with the utterance of certain words or with speaking in certain situations become acute. This causes greater hesitancy, more repetitions, longer prolongations. Thus, a child becomes enmeshed in a problem that keeps feeding itself in an insidious spiralling manner.

### The generalizing effect

Emotional reactions of sufficient intensity to provoke the spiral effect seldom remain confined to the words or situations with which they are first associated. They soon transfer to other words and different situations. This transferring or generalizing of a response to stimuli not exactly the same as the original is explained somewhat differently by different writers. However, there is agreement that

39 What similarities and differences are there in explanations of generalization? What do individual writers mean by *transposition, induction, generalization gradient,* and *partial identity* in connection with transfer of learned responses? See G. Allport, *Personality: A Psychological Interpretation* (New York: Holt, Rinehart and Winston, Inc., 1937), pp. 262-85; B. F. Skinner, *Science and Behavior* (New York: The Macmillan Company, 1953), 132-40; W. Kohler, *Gestalt Psychology* (New York: Liveright Publishing Corp., 1947), 196-208; C. L. Hull, *A Behavior System* (New Haven: Yale University Press, 1952), 167-73; E. K. Hilgard, *Theories of Learning,* 2nd ed. (New York: Appleton-Century-Crofts, Inc., 1956), Chapters 4, 5, and 7.

generalizing seems to occur when an individual discerns elements within new and different situations that are similar to, or possibly identical with, features of situations previously associated with the response. The "elements within new and different situations" may refer to components of the associated response as well as to those of the external environment. In instances of beginning stuttering, the associated response, of course, is the hesitant or fractured utterance of some word. Generalization then may occur when other words are sensed as being similar in some way.

### Transfer of word fear

New or different words offer several possibilities for cues that may serve to cause the transfer. One is a sensed acoustic similarity. Thus, if the spiral effect has resulted in increased difficulty for a child in initiating his first name, say, for example, Michael, he will commence reacting emotionally and experiencing similar trouble on other words with the same beginning sound. At other times, or for some other child, the cue may be the same letter symbol or its alphabet equivalent. Also, words linked with the

> "Gerald," said his mother, "has his worst time with words that begin with a g [dʒi] like his own name. That was one of the first words he stuttered on consistently. Then we began to notice him stuttering on my sister's name, his Aunt Gertrude. And now almost any word that begins with a g [dʒi]seems to give him trouble." We knew this boy had a sister named Janet. Since this word begins with the same *sound* as his first name, we asked whether he had much trouble saying it. We were told that he didn't "unless he's telling me about something she took away from him or something she wouldn't let him do. Then he often stutters on a lot of words."

spiral effect may leave memory traces of tactile or kinesthetic sensations associated with certain contacts or movements of oral structures as they are uttered. When such sensations are experienced in the initiation of new or different words, they, too, conceivably may serve as cues to precipitate more broken speech.

In other instances, cues may be connected to a semantic association; fearful anticipation of trouble spreads to words that have similar meaning. Thus, one stutterer developed an intense fear of the names of states. The generalizing had its origin in an agonizing experience in the sixth grade. "We were studying about the United States. On this particular day we were supposed to give the name of one of the states when she called on us. By the time she got to me, I couldn't think of one that hadn't been mentioned. I got flustered and blurted out one that somebody had already given. So then I had to think of another one. I stuttered pretty bad on that one and all the kids began to titter. It also had been mentioned before. Then I was really flustered and hoped she would go on to somebody else. But she said the class would wait. I finally thought I had one and said 'Mmmmmm . . . . Mmmmmmm . . . . . . Mmmmm-minneapolis.' Everybody roared. I tried to cover my stupid mistake, but I couldn't say the name of the state at all by that time. So the teacher said it for me and then went on. I can't say the name of that state even now without stuttering on it. And ever since then I've had a special fear of the name of any state. They all spell 'trouble' to me. I don't always stutter, but I always think I will."

## Transfer of situation fear

The generalizing of situation fear reflects the same principle. In a new situation, any part that more or less vividly connects it to an earlier one now linked with the spiral effect can generate increased signs of beginning stuttering. Fear of the consequences of talking may transfer, for example, to people who look or sound like someone who previously penalized a child's broken speech. Or it may be the similarity of a place that evokes memories of unpleasant experiences. In the mind of a stutterer, the classroom can remain a chamber of horrors for years. One successful businessman we know has told us that he still seldom talks when he attends the meetings of one organization to which he belongs. "I think it's the armchairs they have in that room at the City Hall where we meet. They're just like the ones we had in school." In any child for whom the spiral effect is beginning to create more obvious signs of stuttering, the generalizing of situation and word fears can quickly multiply the occurrence of broken speech.

## Attempted solutions

The child caught in such a spiralling set of circumstances is driven to seek ways for solving the problem. If the emotional distress is a product of pronounced concern, he will begin trying somehow to *avoid* the now dreaded disruptions. If increasing amounts of frustration are being experienced, his reactions will tend to reflect attempts to *escape* the difficulty encountered in his efforts to utter certain words. Avoidance and escape are the two chief reactions to the anticipation or experience of stuttering.

### *Avoidance Devices*

Avoidance reactions are of three general types. One type consists of attempts to avoid feared words or situations literally and completely. Among the ways a child may try to do this are by (*a*) becoming much less talkative, (*b*) refusing to speak on occasion, (*c*) saying a whole thought in a different way, (*d*) stopping before a feared word and waiting until the listener supplies it, (*e*) substituting a synonym for the one feared, (*f*) speaking in a low voice or mumbling sentences, (*g*) playing sick, (*h*) assuming a special attitude such as a belligerence, confidence, or clowning, and (*i*) pretending not to know the answer to questions. And there are others.

A second type consists of various delaying tactics. Attempts are made to postpone feared situations or the actual utterance of feared words. Postponement devices for situations include pretending not to have heard the question (or the telephone), developing a sudden coughing spell or some other ailment that temporarily prevents talking, and all sorts of excuses for not yet being ready. Occasionally these same reactions are associated with fears of specific words rather than of situations. Another device commonly used in attempts to delay the actual initiation of feared words consists of preceding the word attempts by (*a*) some accessory vocalization ("uh," "er," or "well" is used most frequently), (*b*) a silent pause, or (*c*) repetition of a word or phrase.

The third way in which the stutterer may try to avoid stuttering consists of ritualistic behaviors used to help him actually utter his feared words. Some stutterers seem to feel that if they can just get started, the feared word will be spoken successfully. Here, too, we find a variety of specific devices employed. Accessory vocalization is sometimes used. "Uh" or "er" is spoken as if it were an integral part of the feared word. A child may say, "This is a good . . . . . . . uhbanana" or "Uhcan I have a piece of . . uhpie?" Van Riper (*38:342*) tells of one stutterer named Ranney who always passed as O'Ranney because she used the "Oh" as a device to get started on her name. In some cases, we find extraneous movements being used. Feared words are attempted in time with a sudden jaw jerk, an eyeblink, or a quick hand movement. Others may speak whole series of words preceding the feared ones very rapidly. They sort of race through in an apparent effort to get up enough momentum to carry them right on past the expected trouble. Some begin to take a quick little inhalation just as they get ready to try a feared word. Sometimes the word is then completed on inhaled air. Others try to solve the problem with a sudden change in pitch or intensity as the first part of a word is produced. There are literally hundreds of these ritualistic tricks used to say the feared word without stuttering. Occasionally they work and when this happens the stutterer understandably is inclined to continue to use them.

### *Escape Devices*

The problem is different for the child with whom the spiral effect is associated with pronounced feelings of frustration. His distress is a matter of being in trouble periodically rather than expecting it to occur. He finds himself seemingly trapped into a series of reverberating syllabic repetitions or uncontrollable prolongations. The stutterer feels he must find some way to escape such frustrating experiences. The emotion he feels tends to beget aggressive rather than withdrawal reactions. So this child is most likely to respond by literally trying harder and harder—and again harder—to talk. He tries to force his way forward. He increases the tension in his lips, his tongue, or in the laryngeal area and attempts to "muscle" his way out of the trouble. Often a child will first change the automatized repetitions into prolongations before trying to use greater force. And some react first by interrupting unsuccessful word attempts, by recoiling, and then by beginning again. These children may immediately initiate another direct attack on a troublesome word or, as anger changes to or becomes fused with fear, they may retreat and then try to escape by means of one or more of the devices mentioned earlier for avoiding trouble.

40 For additional information about devices used by stutterers to avoid or escape trouble see C. Van Riper, *Speech Correction, Principles and Methods*, 4th ed. (Englewood Cliffs, N. J.: Prentice-Hall, Inc., 1963), pp. 340-44. How does his classification of devices differ from ours? Utilizing either of them, analyze the behavior patterns from tapes or records of several young stutterers and then compare the results with those of two of your classmates who listened to the same samples.

## THE SOLUTIONS BECOME ADVANCED SYMPTOMS

What happens when a stuttering child tries to solve his problem by means of one or more of these various avoidance or escape devices? He finds some that occasionally appear successful. By their use stuttering is avoided or escaped. The intermittent reinforcement is very potent. Success serves to reinforce the device; so it is used again when trouble occurs or is expected. Unfortunately, all the situations and words that have come to be a part of the spiral effect are not invested with the same degree of emotional distress. Some evoke more than the usual amount of fear or frustration. And when this happens, the child finds himself having to use exaggerated versions of the devices. The one or two utterances of "uh" or "well" that succeeded in the situations of mild stress become three or four or more when the fear is great. The brief pause changes to an extended silence. The slight tensing of lips turns into a pronounced squeezing in an intensified effort to escape from trouble. Stuttering grows.

As it grows its greater abnormality is noted by the listener. Adverse reactions increase. As moments of stuttering become longer and more severe, talking smoothly becomes more difficult. The child who formerly was afraid now has frustration added to his problem. The frustrated child becomes fearful. The spiral effect is amplified and increased by this new abnormality and the new unpleasant feelings. Even the person who at times succeeds in avoiding feared words or situations completely finds he has not solved his problem. Each success unfortunately increases the importance of avoiding trouble the next time. Hence, the fear becomes greater, not less. Stutterers can build up so much fear as a result of successful avoidance of the telephone, for example, that they will tell deliberate lies about calls that came when they were alone. Some have told us about refusing to accept or ask for a second date when they managed to get through the first one without stuttering. Complete avoidance can breed terrifying fears.

As Sheehan (*27*:155) states: "The tragedy of the stutterer's avoidance is not that it always fails, but that it sometimes succeeds."

However much these new elements of the problem may motivate a child to wish he could stop avoiding or get rid of other devices that so often no longer help (they actually make things worse), he finds himself continuing to use them. They become the abnormal, visible, and audible signs of advanced stuttering. Their appearance signifies the beginning of a marked change in the problem that stuttering presents. They indicate that the increasing feelings of fear and frustration are becoming integral features of the problem.

In summary, this advanced stage, characterized by the increasing emotional reactions, more noticeable and frustrating trouble in talking, and a growing feeling that the problem is insoluble, represents a critical phase of stuttering. However, the appearance of these new features does not necessarily indicate the presence of a serious, complicated problem justifying treatment different from that for the beginning stutterer. The earlier patterns still tend to occur frequently. The stuttering continues to fluctuate a great deal. Sieges of trouble are still interspersed with periods of fluency. In most instances the new patterns of behavior do not become fixated for some time. In short, although the behavior patterns are similar if not identical, advanced stuttering and the ultimate stage of this disorder, *secondary* stuttering, are not necessarily synonymous.

## Advanced versus secondary stuttering

WE HAVE EXPLAINED HOW STUTTERING CHANGES AS A CHILD becomes more and more concerned and frustrated by the occurrence of broken speech and his unsuccessful efforts to avoid or escape from the troublesome experiences. And we have said that, even though the stuttering has become more complex and severe, there are times when the difficulty may still not justify its being considered a clinical problem and requiring treatment different from that for the beginning stutterer. The necessity for radically different treatment is not indicated until stuttering becomes

# 4 secondary stuttering as a clinical problem

a *fixed* behavior pattern; until the behavior and the associated emotional reactions have been internalized. This is what changes stuttering from a relatively innocuous disorder to a complex clinical problem. The spiral becomes a self-perpetuating circle. The stuttering becomes its own cause and may then persist independently of original sources. In short, the stuttering behavior attains *functional autonomy*. When, and only when this occurs, can the person be said to be a confirmed or secondary stutterer.

41 G. Allport, *Personality: A Psychological Interpretation* (New York: Holt, Rinehart and Winston, Inc., 1937), pp. 190-212. J. P. Seward, "The Structure of Functional Autonomy," *The American Psychologist*, XVIII (1963), 703-10.

**Summarize the case presented in these references for this specific concept about behavior that persists in the absence of original motives.**

THE FEAR-REDUCTION THEORY

The process by which stuttering becomes fixated is another of the many controversial issues about the disorder. One highly regarded explanation among speech pathologists is the fear-reduction theory or hypothesis. The concept is predicated on the belief that the normal individual finds intense emotional distress very difficult to endure. Hence, when it is experienced, most people are motivated to get rid of it or at least to have it reduced to a tolerable level. Anything that succeeds in accomplishing this tends to be used again in later situations and eventually becomes an established behavior pattern that cannot easily be terminated. Smoking, in addition to being a pertinent example of functional autonomy, may illustrate the fear-reduction theory. A person may begin smoking as a teenager to avoid being considered immature. But lighting another cigarette gradually becomes an habitual reaction to tension caused by anxiety or fear no longer associated necessarily with the earlier source. And some people even when threatened by cancer or heart trouble find it impossible to stop smoking. It is too firmly embedded as a way of temporarily reducing troublesome emotional tension.

Fear-reduction theory in a similar fashion may explain stuttering. As we have pointed out, intense feelings of

42 For the original theoretical design in connection with stuttering, see G. J. Wischner, "Stuttering Behavior and Learning: A Preliminary Theoretical Formulation," *Journal of Speech and Hearing Disorders,* XV (1950), 324-35.

For evidence in support of the theory from studies of stuttering, see J. Sheehan, "A Conflict Theory of Stuttering," in *Stuttering: A Symposium,* ed. J. Eisenson (New York: Harper & Row, Publishers, Inc., 1958), pp. 132-35.

For information about broader applications of the theory to maladaptive behavior, see B. McCandless, *Children and Adolescents* (New York: Holt, Rinehart and Winston, Inc., 1961), pp. 153-58.

concern or frustration drive a child to seek ways of avoiding or escaping from the broken speech that becomes the focus of his distress. Then, whatever he does that makes it unnecessary to talk, or to use a specific word, or that terminates in the utterance of a troublesome word, results in an immediate mitigation of the emotional turmoil. Thus, in spite of its abnormality and the additional problems it creates, the "stuttering" behavior is reinforced by its success in reducing the unpleasant emotion. Unfortunately, the relief is temporary. The fear, thus fed, grows stronger. The fearful young stutterer now must stutter more or work harder to avoid talking in order to obtain relief from his fear of stuttering! The new behavior becomes automatic, self-perpetuating, and, in many cases, very tenacious.

43 Contrast this interpretation with information in H. Luper, "Consistency of Stuttering in Relation to the Goal Gradient Hypothesis," *Journal of Speech and Hearing Disorders,* XXI (1956), 336-42, in J. G. Sheehan, P. A. Cortese and R. G. Hadley, "Guilt, Shame, and Tension in Graphic Projections of Stuttering," *Journal of Speech and Hearing Disorders,* XXVII (1962), 129-43, and in G. H. Shames and C. E. Sherrick, "A Discussion of Nonfluency and Stuttering as Operant Behavior," *Journal of Speech and Hearing Disorders,* XXVIII (1963), 3-18.

## ADVANCED PATTERNS AS SECONDARY REWARDS

Some authorities, particularly those who view the disorder as a form of neurosis, believe stuttering becomes intrenched because of the secondary neurotic profit it provides. Glauber (*13:*110), for example, tells us, "Stuttering, like any other symptom, is capable of giving a secondary gain—a satisfaction, almost always unconscious, derived from a symptom after it is formed and apart from the deeper satisfaction that caused it to form." He continues with an example: "A surgeon once remarked to a colleague that his patients, especially the women who admired him very much, referred to his stutter as cute. He, it might be noted, was not in treatment." We recall a similar example, a college girl who we thought had been very successful in solving her stuttering problem. She later wrote that she was getting along all right except when she went out with any fellow she did not especially like. Whenever that occurred, she told us she would "stutter all over the place so he wouldn't ask me out again."

Others may find stuttering an effective way of gaining and holding the listener's attention. Or it may become a means of enjoying preferential treatment at home or at school. The implied pity may be hated, but the special

44 J. B. Rotter, *Social Learning and Clinical Psychology* (Englewood Cliffs, N. J.: Prentice-Hall, Inc., 1954), pp. 145-48. In what ways did Robert find his stuttering useful? What is this writer's view of stuttering?

attention can provide more than enough compensating satisfaction for an individual who has pronounced unfulfilled needs for recognition and affection. In other cases, it may become an habitual alibi for failure, or for not trying because of expected failure. In still others, stuttering may come to symbolize repressed hostility and associated feelings of guilt, as Abbott (*1*:428-30) has shown. He can punish his listener and get by scot free. In other cases, the gain lies in the self-punishment the speaker inflicts upon himself when he stutters. It helps him atone for the guilt feelings he has about his hostility towards the listener.

### Self-concept integration

Another explanation for the adhesive quality of secondary stuttering is suggested by the self-concept construct. Accordingly, as a child grows, he is continually acquiring and modifying ideas about himself and the world in which he lives. Eventually he has a confirmed set of ideas, both favorable and unfavorable, logical and illogical, that tend to persist in spite of experiences indicating that his conclusions may be erroneous. Sullivan (32) views this set of ideas, the unitary self-concept, as being composed of numerous images, perpetuated because the associated behavior represents the most satisfactory solution to a given situation available to the individual at the moment. Any disturbance of the self-concept is considered threatening to one's well being. Hence, behavior that persists in creating problems and thus serves to enhance a negative facet of the self-concept is as easily perpetuated as any that reinforce positive aspects. And once an idea about oneself becomes an integral part of the self-concept, the behavior that symbolizes it gets rewarded. Examples abound. The person who continues to think of himself as stupid in spite of his Phi Beta Kappa key; the criminal who cannot be rehabilitated because he's convinced of his "badness"; the individual who denies the accuracy of medical charts about height and weight and still claims he is too fat; these are legion. Similarly, the child who has internalized the idea of being a stutterer may continue stuttering because he's convinced "this is me"; "a stutterer is what I am"; "I couldn't be me and not stutter."

**45** How is this idea supported in S. S. Zelen, J. G. Sheehan, and J. F. T. Bugental, "Self-Perceptions in Stuttering," *Journal of Clinical Psychology*, X (1954), 70-72?

### Understanding the Secondary Stutterer

Regardless of the process by which stuttering behavior becomes fixed and self-perpetuating, the problem presented by the secondary stutterer in most instances is more than troubled talking. Secondary stuttering as a clinical problem tends to have multiple facets or features. There are innumerable possibilities, since chronic stuttering cannot avoid becoming superimposed upon whatever else a stutterer is or does or believes himself to be. A precise and accurate list of all the features of secondary stuttering is impossible to present. The personalities and other attributes of people who stutter simply vary too much. So, also, do their individual reactions to different stresses and differing environments.

A second important aspect of secondary stuttering as a clinical problem is that, although we find the same features in many stutterers, they vary widely in their significance for therapy. A prominent feature for one may have little or no clinical significance for another. Guilt feelings, for example, may be a highly important feature of one stutterer's problem but not of another's. Similarly, one stutterer comes for help only because others have forced him to do so; another seeks his own therapy despite the opposition of his family. When such differences in the individual features of the clinical problem exist, differences in treatment must necessarily follow. There can be no one treatment for stuttering.

The possible *combinations* of component features in terms of their relative significance for therapy are many. Indeed, these new attributes appear, subside, change. A given stutterer may have several behavioral patterns of stuttering, using one for mildly feared situations and another for those full of panic. The relative importance of all behavioral features or patterns cannot always be discerned before therapy is begun. In view of these observations we need not wonder that secondary stuttering is so difficult to understand and to treat. We need not be surprised to discover that any of the many specific treatment methods, applied in the same ways to groups of stutterers, work successfully with some but fail miserably with others. Clinically, no two cases of secondary stuttering present the same problem.

The implications seem obvious. Secondary stuttering is a highly individualized problem so far as therapy is concerned. There are at least three major reasons for this. First, the stuttering may have had a multiple origin in one or more of several different conditions or circumstances; second, chronic stuttering affects people in different ways and to different degrees and becomes an individually defined problem; and lastly, there exist significant individual differences in temperaments, motivation, intelligence, and environments, both past and present. Hence, although common features and patterns among cases allow most stutterers to profit to some extent from a common regime, treatment sooner or later must reflect the differences. In short, to understand the secondary stutterer, we cannot assume that the fact of the stuttering itself defines his problem and indicates the therapy he needs. The form and frequency and severity of the stuttering may not be ignored, of course, but we must also understand the *kind* of problem the stutterer possesses and the kind of person who possesses the stuttering. This requires identification of the significant features of the stuttering as well as of the stutterer.

This is a difficult task. Tests and other diagnostic procedures have not yet been developed to provide the information the speech therapist so often needs. The needed skill in judgment usually can be gained only by experience. And even the most experienced therapists must always work in the foggy atmosphere of uncertainty. To help you get started, the best we can do is to provide some information about those features and patterns which clinical experience has led us to believe are presented most often and to explain how they may determine the emphasis or the kind of therapy. The best way we know to do this is by citing some illustrative cases.

### *Karen*

Karen, a college freshman, was obviously nervous and embarrassed. She sat tensely in a chair, moving her hands, alternately grasping one with the other, and looking down or out of a window at our back. She had been referred to us by the instructor of her class in public speaking. We said we understood she was having a little difficulty with her speech in that class. She spoke in a low voice with a noticeable lack of animation.

"Oh, well, some . . . . . . sometimes, I guess. But it doesn't . . it doesn't . . . . . . you know bother me."
"Do you have similar difficulty in other classes?"
"Not uh . . . well very often. I don't re . . . . re . . . uh . . you know uhtalk in my other classes. I'm too busy takin' uh . . uhyou know uh notes, writin' stuff down."
"Did you used to recite in high school classes?"
"Some . . . . sometimes. I really didn't have to re . . . to talk in class. I got good uh . . you know . . . . good grades anyway."
"Have you had help of any kind for your speech?"
"No."
"Have you ever wanted any help for it?"
"No . . . uh . . uh well . . . well maybe, sometimes. Most of the time I just . . . well . . just hoped it would . . . . . would dis . . . you know, go away."
"It has bothered you at times?"
"Well, no. I never . . . . well . . . . you know let it bother me. I just don't uh . . . don't think about it."
"Do your parents ever say anything about it?"
"Oh, no, they uh . . . uh . . . no, they don't."
"Do you ever have any trouble with your speech when you talk to them?"

"Some . . . sometimes. But they . . they . . . uh . . they never say anything."

"Have you ever been teased about it by any of the kids at school?"

"No. Well, not . . . . not uh . . you know for a long time."

"Did you have a lot of close friends in high school?"

"Uh . . uh . . . well, enough."

"Did you sometimes wish you had more?"

"Some . . . sometimes."

"Is reading aloud any special problem for you?"

"Yes. I . . . I . . I uhdon't ever do that unless I . . I . . . . well . . . you know unless I have to."

"How did you happen to get into the speech class?"

"Well, the uh . . . the uhadviser, well, he just put me in . . . . in the class."

"Was that a course you really wanted to take?"

"No, but I didn't . . . . . well . . . . you know want to say anything."

"Are you interested in any help now for your speech?"

"Uh . . . uh . . . . uhwell, I don't really think I need any. Would I have to . . . . . . have to . . . well . . . . . you know, uhcome over here to this place?"

We told her she would, but hastened to assure her that no one was going to force her to take part in the clinic program. She then wanted to know what she would have to do if she came to the clinic, how we would go about trying to help her. We explained the general aims of the therapy and then suggested she get the details by talking with another girl who had been through the program the previous year and was still on the campus. The meeting was arranged and about two weeks later the former case came to the clinic with Karen in tow.

We find many stutterers like Karen. They do not all

46 E. Douglass and B. Quarrington, "The Differentiation of Interiorized and Exteriorized Stuttering," *Journal of Speech and Hearing Disorders*, XVII (1952), 377-85.

**How would these writers classify Karen as a stutterer? Make a list of the distinguishing features.**

reveal their problems in the same way. Some have more trouble, some have less. Some are more willing to admit a need for help; others are less so. However, for all of this breed, the problem which stuttering has come to represent is dominated by feelings of shame, embarrassment, and sometimes guilt. These people feel they cannot afford to have their stuttering recognized. The more severe cases view stuttering as a shameful curse. Hence, they work arduously and at times desperately to keep it hidden. Karen succeeded most of the time (she thought) by the use of "uh," "well," and "you know," by substituting, and by presenting logical reasons for not talking in some situations. Also, by speaking in a low voice, she further minimized the chance that any stuttering would be noticed. Other stutterers like Karen reveal a variety of similar devices, all having the same purpose: the avoidance of identification as a stutterer.

These cases also reveal wide variation in the depth of their feelings of shame, embarrassment, and guilt. For some, the feelings are fairly superficial. They are close to the surface, and prove to be easily verbalized. Others simply cannot endure any discussion of their stuttering problem. For them, disclosure, exposure is far too painful. Some of these people never succeed in becoming able to seek professional help. They nurse their shame as they hide it.

These stutterers vary in still another way. They differ in their abilities to accept the stuttering label and in their tolerances for fluency disruptions. Some simply cannot bear the stigma of the word. The word has become a symbol of shame. They cannot stand having it applied to them. For these individuals, a major part of their problem is truly semantic. Karen proved to be such a case. We learned from her parents that the stuttering *never* had been discussed within the family nor was it allowed to be mentioned by anyone else. They had thought any direct admission of the problem could have only dire results, that it would cause her to become too self-conscious about it. The result was that Karen came to believe that stuttering must be something too horrible to talk about. As soon as she understood her parents' behavior, Karen became more willing to stutter openly and she soon made the happy discovery that other people (to whom she had generalized her interpretation of her parents' reactions?) were not shocked or revolted to learn that she stuttered. In fact, much to her surprise, she discovered that nearly everyone who knew her had known it all along.

We find others among these cases who are willing to allow themselves to be called stutterers *so long as their speech is free of any recognizable stuttering*. These people accept the label and most will fluently admit to being stutterers. However, they reveal a notable reluctance to allow any stuttering to occur. And they seldom care to be identified with stutterers who actually do stutter. They are usually poor candidates for group therapy.

The attitudes of a third group of these cases combine the features of the other two. These are the stutterers who can neither tolerate the label (or any substitute such as nonfluency) nor bear to have any fluency breaks in their speech. These people have a highly distorted idea of normal fluency. They tend to be seeking perfect speech. Anything short of absolute fluency is stuttering, they feel, and thus will be a continual source of embarrassment.

### *Basic Treatment Needs*

The first (and frequently the greatest) need of stutterers like Karen should be obvious. They must have help for the

47 In the context of this section, evaluate the treatment for stuttering described in W. Johnson et. al., *Speech Handicapped School Children*, rev. ed. (New York: Harper & Row, Publishers, Inc., 1956), 283-93; D. E. Williams, "A Point of View about Stuttering," *Journal of Speech and Hearing Disorders*, XXII (1957), 390-97; O. Bloodstein, "Stuttering as an Anticipatory Struggle Reaction," in *Stuttering: A Symposium*, ed. J. Eisenson (New York: Harper & Row, Publishers, Inc., 1958), pp. 40-52; B. Bryngelson, "Stuttering and Personality Development," *Nervous Child*, II (1943), 219-23.

covert features of their problem: the feelings of shame, embarrassment, and, when present, guilt. These cases cannot be expected to talk freely or do anything else constructive about their stuttering until we have helped them explore and test the validity of their feelings. They must be helped to discover the extent to which their fears are justified. Occasionally, when such a case finds he has been operating on a false premise and becomes willing to attack his feared words directly, he discovers that there is little if anything left of his problem. The dreaded stuttering doesn't occur. He becomes a normally fluent person. These cases are good examples of Johnson's (Search Item No. 47, p. 216) concise definition: ". . . stuttering is what a speaker does trying not to stutter again."

More often than not, however, when these cases begin to cease their avoidance devices, they reveal more obvious evidence of difficulty in uttering many of their feared words. They block. They show some struggle behavior. Tremors may appear. Concerning this development, Douglass and Quarrington (Search Item No. 46, p. 380) have this to say: "It is perhaps an observation of some significance that the stuttered speech pattern of the interiorized stutterer when it does appear is of a catastrophic nature. Although comparatively short in duration, it is intense in severity and might be described as a 'true' spasm, that is, an involuntary muscular disruption, rapidly clonic in nature and usually confined to the sound that is being uttered." When this feature of the problem emerges, we must be ready to help the case find a solution. Otherwise, we should not be surprised if our stutterer retreats to his avoidance and disguising devices and stubbornly resists our efforts to help him.

**48** **Describe and explain three common forms of resistance. See O. Bloodstein (No. 47, 55-58).**

*Joe*

All secondary stutterers probably harbor some feelings of shame and embarrassment and at times utilize devices to hide evidence of their difficulty. However, there are many for whom those features have little significance so far as therapy is concerned. Instead, the problem stuttering has come to represent is dominated by some different combination of features. The case we now present illustrates one of these different patterns.

Joe was a sixteen-year-old high-school student with an IQ of 136. He was sophisticated, outspoken, and very verbal, though he stuttered severely and frequently. He seldom spoke a complete sentence without trouble on several words. The stuttering was so effortful that at times his face flushed with the struggle, not from embarrassment. His stuttering was about the same in frequency and explosive severity when he read aloud as when he just talked. It was reduced only slightly through three readings of the same paragraph. He told us, "About the only time I don't stutter is when I'm talking to my dog."

The actual initiation of feared words beginning with plosives was usually followed by a noticeable contorting of his whole face. On words beginning with certain continuants, he would prolong the sound, sometimes for as long as he had air left in his lungs. He struggled rather fiercely in his efforts to talk. Still, he appeared unafraid to talk to anyone—strangers, authority figures, anyone. He seldom let his stuttering stop him from speaking, and there were few subjects about which he felt he didn't know enough to have something to say. Some would consider him brash. He said his stuttering was always a problem to him and he freely admitted it was a source of embarrassment. "Of course it's embarrassing," he said. "I don't think anyone could stutter like I do and not be embarrassed by it. But I haven't been able to stop it and, frankly, I like to talk."

He had taken part in many school activities of a social nature. He had been president of his sophomore class and had spoken briefly to assemblies on a few occasions. He enjoyed being a leader. His ambition was to be a surgeon, "but I may change my mind and go into politics."

The etiology of his stuttering was obscure. He said he guessed he had been stuttering since he began to talk. "That's what my parents have always said, anyway. I know I've been stuttering for as long as I can remember." Joe was an only child, born when his parents were in their early thirties. His father was an engineering consultant. "He's an engineer's engineer, if you know what I mean. He goes all over the country on important projects and my mother and I often go with him in the summer. I've gotten to meet a lot of important people that way. My parents never made me feel that my stuttering embarrassed them. I suppose that's why I've never been as embarrassed about it as other stutterers are. I just say what I have to say whether I stutter or not and if it bothers somebody, well, that's just too damn bad."

He had had therapy on three different occasions before he came to see us. The first occurred during the third grade when he was enrolled in the school's speech-correction program. "She tried to get me to relax. It didn't work. I refused to go the next year and my parents didn't argue about it. Then I went to a camp the summer before I went into the eighth grade. It was my own idea. I wrote and got information about a lot of different places. It was fun, but I didn't get any help there either. They worked a lot on our attitudes about our stuttering and tried to help us become adjusted to our fears. It helped some of the stutterers a lot, I thought, but not me." When he was a sophomore, a speech therapist was assigned to his high school. Joe decided to take advantage of that opportunity. He went twice a week during that school year. There usually were two or three other stutterers at each meeting. "There was more about becoming objective and overcoming our fears. Hell, I'm not afraid. I just get stuck. Then I have to do all these crazy things to get myself unstuck. It burns me up. I hate it, I really do. It makes me so damn mad that I can't stop it. I sure hope you got something that will really help."

Here is a much different pattern of prominent features. The stuttering is obvious. We find few indications of attempts to hide or deny it as a problem. The associated emotions are frustration, anger, and hostility. Here again, among the stutterers who represent this pattern of behavior and attitudes, we can expect to encounter great variety in the forms and in the severity of the stuttering. Also, we shall find some who reveal more pronounced feelings of embarrassment (commonly manifested in an averting of the eyes from the listener's face during moments of stuttering). Others, because of uncomfortable guilt feelings, are less willing to reveal their anger and hostility. We also may note the use of substitutions, starters, and recoil and retrial devices among these people. But they keep communicating—at times compulsively.

With Joe and others like him, the distinguishing features lie in the form of the stuttering itself and the related attitudes. These people seldom detour or back away from feared words or situations. Instead, they attack them, head on. They wrestle with their mysterious adversary. In the process, they may gasp, choke, snort, protrude their tongues, jerk their jaws, their heads, their arms, their legs. Eyes may be squeezed or the whole face contorted in the desperate struggle to talk. The severe cases seldom present a pretty picture. At times the picture is truly shocking. Such behavior, in a person who has no known physical ailment and who at times can say any word perfectly, may impress the beginning therapist not only as strange and unusual but as senseless and unnecessary.

The impression contains an element of truth. No individual necessarily must stutter in a particular way. How he stutters is due to how he learned to stutter. However, when stutterers like Joe come to us for help, it is very important that we appreciate their felt inability to prevent the stoppage or the struggling that occurs at times when they try to utter some word. These people tend to feel helpless when they stutter. Many, like Joe, claim they "just get stuck." And they are convinced there is nothing they can do about it at that moment. Others describe the experience as a feeling of a sudden loss of control over their tongues or their mouths. It is seldom possible to help such stutterers by having them note the nonfluencies of normal speakers or by pointing out the complete freedom from trouble they, themselves, have on many occasions. Indeed, for many, vivid perception of their own fluency may be responsible for a significant additional ingredient of their distress. It makes them feel stupid as well as helpless.

One other common aspect of this feature of the problem presented by these cases deserves mention at this time. We refer to the lack of knowledge many of them have about what is happening when they stutter. It would be reasonable to suppose that people whose stuttering is out in the open, so to speak, and for whom embarrassment, though present, is not an outstanding feature of their problem, should be quite aware of their behavior when they stutter. Such is seldom the case, however. Beyond being highly conscious of some bizarre mannerism such as a violent head jerk or a pronounced tremor, few have more than a vague idea about what they actually do when they stutter. Sometime during the course of the problem, these people tend to alienate themselves from the stuttering behavior. In fact, during the moment of stuttering, they may not see or hear anything. One man reported, "I'm absolutely blind and deaf to my environment during the stuttering block." Accordingly, being confronted with their

49 E. Froeschels and R. Rieber, "The Problem of Auditory and Visual Imperceptivity in Stutterers," *Folia Phoniatrica*, XV (1963), 13-20. What is meant by "transitory articulatory monomania?" If embarrassment is not a prominent feature of the problem presented by the case whose stuttering consists principally of overt blocking, how may such a reaction be explained? How might the implications of this study be researched further?

stuttering behavior can be as much of a traumatic experience for many of these cases as it is for those who hide their stuttering. Therapists who utilize tape recorders and mirrors in their work with stutterers must exercise considerable caution in the use of these and similar treatment aids with these people.

### *Basic Treatment Needs*

Stutterers like Joe seldom respond well to therapies that

50 In the context of this section, evaluate the treatment for stuttering described in C. Van Riper, "Experiments in Stuttering Therapy," in *Stuttering: A Symposium*, ed. J. Eisenson (New York: Harper & Row, Publishers, Inc., 1958), Chapter 6.

emphasize personality evaluation, semantic reorientation, or other methods of emotional readjustment in the initial phases of treatment. Their first and occasionally their only needs are for more appropriate and normal methods of attacking feared words and a more efficient and effective way of extricating themselves when they feel blocked.

There are many techniques employed by speech therapists to help stutterers accomplish these two things. Among them are negative practice, rate control, relaxation, both general and differential, voluntary stuttering, easy repetition or the "bounce" method, cancellation, pull-outs, "chewing speech," and preparatory sets. Any may be

51 For details about these and other similar techniques, see:

J. Eisenson, "A Perserverative Theory of Stuttering," in *Stuttering: A Symposium*, ed. J. Eisenson (New York: Harper & Row, Publishers, Inc., 1958), pp. 261-64.

O. Bloodstein, *Stuttering for Professional Workers* (Chicago: National Society for Crippled Children and Adults, 1959), pp. 65-79.

K. Dunlap, "Stammering: Its Nature, Etiology and Therapy," *Journal of Comparative Psychology*, XXXVII (1944), 187-202.

C. Van Riper, "Symptomatic Therapy for Stuttering," in *Handbook of Speech Pathology*, ed. L. E. Travis (New York: Appleton-Century-Crofts, Inc., 1957), Chapter 27.

C. Van Riper, "The Treatment of Stuttering," *Speech*, XVII (1953), 17-20. E. Froeschels, "Pathology and Therapy of Stuttering," *The Nervous Child*, II (1942), 146-61.

F. Brook, *Stammering and Its Treatment* (London: Pitman Medical Publishing Co., 1957), Chapters 4, 5, 6, and 7.

successfully utilized by individual stutterers. However, according to West (*40*:217) and to Bloodstein (No. 50, p. 56), any technique to eliminate or control stuttering which is taught only as a form of distraction seldom provides more than temporary relief. As soon as the distractive value is dissipated, the old fears return and, with them, the stuttering. Satisfactory results are obtained, in most instances, only when the learned technique is able to serve as an acceptable substitute for or method of control over the stuttering in at least the majority of situations in which it is needed. Few stutterers will continue long to use any technique for eliminating or controlling stuttering that turns out either to be ineffective in stressful situations or to consist of some mannerism or form of talking no more desirable than their stuttering.

### *Lloyd*

Another sizable group of cases presents a third fairly distinct combination of features. To illustrate the general form of the stuttering found among those who represent this pattern, we shall attempt to describe the speech of thirteen-year-old Lloyd. He is talking about a vacation trip.

> "W . . W . Well, fff . . . fr . . fr . . . ffirst . . . first we . . . we . . uh . . w . . we went tt . . tt . . t . tto NN . . . NNN . . . NNew York . . NNew York. I . . I . . . I g . . g . . . g (each attempt on this sound was accompanied by a brief gutteral "uh") g . . . g . got to see . . . ss . . . sss . ssssee the YY . . Y . . . YYankees plll . . pll (on these initiations of the word *play,* there was some slight but noticeable tension and mild tremors in the lip area) plll . . . p . play b . . . . b . . b . . . . ball" (again we could hear a brief gutteral "uh" on each of the aborted utterances of the initial sound in this last word, but there was no obvious struggling, and the word was uttered with no discernible difficulty).

This boy talked and stuttered about as freely as Joe, yet there was a marked hesitancy in his behavior. The pattern of disrupted fluency presented by stutterers like Lloyd appears to reflect more of an unwillingness to keep moving forward than an apparent inability to do so. These people give the impression of proceeding with great caution through words and sentences. There is ambivalence and abulia in their oral communication behavior. They begin sentences or words, then flinch and recoil from sensed or expected trouble. And in the frequent repetitions and retrials, there is little evidence of any real effort in the utterances. They are like a person who must cross a frozen lake, but fears the ice won't hold. Every step is taken cautiously, tentatively, after carefully testing the ice ahead.

Again, we wish to remind the reader about the variations in the frequency and the specific ways of stuttering that he can expect to find among the cases who represent any general pattern. Within this particular group, there are some who have very little overt trouble in talking beyond the first sentence or two of a paragraph or a complete thought. Once started, these cases speak fluently unless interrupted by the listener. Others may stutter noticeably only when explaining something (especially their own behavior or ideas) or when they are forced to clarify an explanation.

The dominant emotion encountered most frequently in stutterers like Lloyd is anxiety. These cases are more or less bedeviled by general feelings of apprehension and foreboding. Most of them harbor pronounced feelings of insecurity and inadequacy. And, although stuttering is often the perceived or at least the stated source of their misery, it seldom is the only cause. These people usually reveal a history of additional development problems. Lloyd, for example, though never a sickly child, had always been on the frail side in physique. "He never could keep up with the other boys," his mother reported. "He always seemed to be the first one to get hurt. When they played hide and seek, he'd fall over a wagon or a railing. When they played soldiers or cops and robbers, he'd get hit in the face with a stick or stumble and fall down the ravine where they always played. He was never seriously hurt, but I was forever patching him up. It never seemed to bother him too much. He'd get banged up and cry for awhile and then be right back out playing the same games again. He got better as he got older, but he still isn't too strong or well coordinated. Just last year he went out for basketball. They let him stay on the team, but he only got to play a few minutes and he wasn't encouraged to go back this year. We try to make him eat more, and I make him take vitamin tablets, but he's always been so sensitive about his size and weight that I try not to nag him too much."

Lloyd also was slow in learning to talk and to read. His mother stated that he didn't begin talking until after his third birthday. However, ". . . once he got started, he soon talked as well as the other children his age." Learning to read didn't occur as spontaneously. "He was smart enough in other ways, but he couldn't read at all well until he was in the sixth grade. We have supposed that his stuttering had a lot to do with it, but then he didn't stutter too much until the third grade, so maybe it was just the other way around. We never have known what got him started to stutter. It went in streaks for a long time. Sometimes he'd go for a month or two without any trouble at all. We really didn't pay any special attention to it until after he was in the fourth grade, and even then my husband and I thought he would still outgrow it. We were more concerned about his reading than his stuttering. He still isn't a good reader. He has to spend a lot of time on his assignments. But he won't let his father or me help him. He goes to his older sister when he gets stuck. Sometimes we think Lloyd believes we are partial to his younger brother. I suppose I have picked on him more, but it certainly isn't because we think less of him. He's just been more of a problem. I've always had to be warning him to be careful.

I don't think I'm the nervous type, but I have had to worry more about Lloyd. I've always been afraid that he would be hurt seriously sometime."

### *Basic Treatment Needs*

The therapist who presents an unusually friendly and

52 In the context of this section, particularly for the age group represented by Lloyd, evaluate the treatment approach described in B. Bryngelson, M. E. Chapman, and O. K. Hansen, *Know Yourself—A Workbook for Those Who Stutter* (Minneapolis: Burgess, 1944), and in M. E. Chapman, *Self-Inventory,* 3rd ed. (Minneapolis: Burgess, 1959).

reassuring manner to cases like Lloyd is sometimes pleasantly surprised with the rapid change in the stuttering. Some of these stutterers become completely fluent in the clinic situation in a relatively short time. And occasionally, when neither the stuttering nor the anxiety is pronounced, the fluency transfers to other situations. Usually, however, the freedom from stuttering experienced in the presence of a likeable therapist does not extend very far beyond the door of the therapy room. The majority of these cases need more than the temporary feelings of greater confidence acquired from a few sessions with an accepting and reassuring therapist. Some need a great deal of help with the overt stuttering which is uncovered when they become willing and able to inhibit the repetitions and retrials. Stoppages and struggle behavior is revealed on many words. Genuine tremors may appear. We cannot expect these cases to be willing to give up their less troublesome and possibly less noticeable stuttering without helping them find a more tolerable way of uttering their feared words.

The treatment for others among this group must be more squarely aimed at the underlying sources of the anxiety which is serving to precipitate and perpetuate the stuttering behavior. The positive effects, if any, of speech

53 For a relevant example, see M. B. Jensen, "A Case of Extreme Language Disability Concealed by Stuttering," *Journal of Clinical Psychology,* XIV (1948), 93-96.

therapy alone are limited and usually temporary. These stutterers must be helped to find solutions for other felt deficiencies. As long as they feel anxious and apprehensive about their appearance, their reading ability, their athletic skills, or any other real or imagined undesirable difference, these cases seldom are able to overcome their ambivalent and halfhearted behavior when they talk. They have too much fear of being unfavorably evaluated as individuals, not as just stutterers. They must keep watching to be sure it is safe to go ahead. They expect the roof to fall in at any moment.

With these cases, the stuttering is more understandable when viewed as a symptom of underlying anxiety about other things than as a learned reaction pattern to developed concern or sensed difficulty with speech. Effective treatment may need to include some direct work with the stuttering, but the emphasis must be on the dominant emotional feature and the factors that created and/or are continuing to keep the anxiety alive.

### *Carl*

We have described three different patterns of stuttering behavior and presented some information about the problem the behavior tends to represent in each instance. We have seen how cases like Karen attempt to solve their felt difficulty in talking by avoiding feared situations and words, or by disguising or trying to ignore the fact of their stuttering. Others, like Joe, are not markedly inclined to avoid situations and they plunge headlong into their feared words. Those in a third group, represented by Lloyd, tend to react to sensed or expected trouble by recoiling, by beginning again one or more times, and in general, by speaking their way through sentences in a manner similar to the cautious and hesitant progress of a person walking barefooted along a beach littered with invisible pieces of broken glass.

There is yet another pattern of prominent and clinically significant features often presented by secondary stutterers. Some cases confronted with the necessity for uttering their feared words do not resort to deception or struggle or retrials. Instead, they give up. They quit. They surrender. Meet twenty-eight-year-old Carl. When asked to tell us his first name, he proceeded to assume what appeared to be the proper tongue placement for the first sound and then, with his mouth fixed in a half-open posture, silently and with complete passivity looked at us for an estimated ten seconds. Nothing connected with the utterance of his name beyond the appropriate initial posturing appeared to be happening. No sound, no movement, no struggle, no observable tremor. Nothing. He finally broke the trancelike silence, shifted around in his chair, swallowed, then assumed the previously described oral posture and we looked at each other in complete silence for another eight or ten seconds. A dropped pin could have been heard. Suddenly, Carl again shifted around in his chair and shattered the silence by saying, with no trouble whatsoever, "I'm sure having an awful time just saying my name." We nodded a yes. He went to work on it once more. This time, during the extended silence, he occasionally would frown and we could note a hint of effort. Finally, he spoke again. "I-I-I-I-I (as he prolonged the utterance of this word, his face had a sad, pained look. His voice rose to a whimper.) -I-I-I cccccan't say it, I g . . . . g . . guess. CCCCCCCCCarl . . . . Carl. Yeah, there. N . . . N . . Now it's easy."

This man's speech was filled with those long silent pauses and extended prolongations when he talked, which was not often. He had managed to acquire a college degree, a wife, and a baby, but the only job he had been able to get was doing repair work in the back room of a television and radio store. He had a long history of unsuccessful therapy, including psychiatric treatment on two occasions. He claimed these were ineffective because he could not talk enough and it became too expensive. Three different speech therapists had worked with him, one over a period of three of the five years he spent in college. In each instance, he had gotten much better, but had been unable to retain the benefits of the treatments. "I can always do well after I've been around a clinic for awhile. I've even given talks to speech-correction classes and been able to demonstrate various methods for controlling my stuttering. Twice I was almost completely fluent for several months. Then I went bad during the summer vacations. I don't know what it is. I guess I just don't have enough confidence in myself. I know that whenever I do feel confident, I don't stutter much. But it doesn't last. I know I should be able to lick this thing. I've sure had enough help. But I just can't seem to do it on my own. . . . I've got to whip it so I can get a decent job. . . . But I've tried so many times already. . . . I really don't know. Maybe I should just throw in the towel.

The last sentence, revealing Carl's attitude of resigna-

54 What is said about this feature of stuttering in D. A. Barbara, *Stuttering: A Psychodynamic Approach To Its Understanding and Treatment?* (New York: The Julian Press, 1954), Chapter 15.

tion, was said in jest, but we believe it also contained a plea for help that was no joke. Stutterers like Carl have little strength for solving their stuttering or any other problem that besets them. They are plagued by feelings of impotence and worthlessness. They seem foredoomed to fail at everything they try. Stuttering does not make these people feel just helpless. For them, the situation is utterly hopeless. They often feel frustrated by their trouble in talking, but any anger or hostility is turned inward. They seek and accept help for their problem, then hate themselves a little more for their weakness.

In the case histories of these stutterers, we often find evidence of overprotection or rejection to account for the feelings of self-doubt, weakness, and guilt. In Carl's case, we learned from a written autobiography that his mother had lost her other two children at birth and had so much trouble with his birth that she was advised to have no more. Unfortunately for Carl, she apparently had hoped that the baby she did not lose would be a girl. He wrote that he could remember being reminded about this on many occasions.

The parents separated when Carl was five years old. He said his mother told him she thought that was when his stuttering began. His mother had to go to work, and for the next five years, they lived with a spinster relative. About her, Carl wrote, "I don't believe she ever liked kids, period." Then his mother married a widower who had two young daughters. As soon as he got through high school, Carl joined the army. He remembered hearing his mother say, just before he left, "If you were a girl now, you could get married and wouldn't have to go into the army."

### *Basic Treatment Needs*

We could have provided Carl with another temporary

55 In the context of this section, evaluate and compare the treatment approaches in:

L. E. Travis, "The Unspeakable Feelings of People, with Special Reference to Stuttering," in *Handbook of Speech Pathology,* ed. L. E. Travis (New York: Appleton-Century-Crofts, Inc., 1957), pp. 927-45.

I. P. Glauber, "The Psychoanalysis of Stuttering," in *Stuttering: A Symposium,* ed. J. Eisenson (New York: Harper & Row, Publishers, Inc., 1958), pp. 110-18.

C. H. Miller, "Psychotherapy in Action: A Case Report," in *The Psychotherapy of Stuttering,* ed. D. A. Barbara (Springfield, Ill.: C. C. Thomas, 1962), Chapter 10.

C. R. Rogers, *Counseling and Psychotherapy* (New York: Houghton Mifflin, 1942), 261-437.

R. F. Hejna, *Speech Disorders and Nondirective Therapy* (New York: Ronald Press, 1960), 97-329.

J. Seeman, *The Case of Jim* (Nashville, Tenn.: Educational Test Bureau, 2106 Pierce Ave., 1957).

For an interesting discussion of the role of insight in psychotherapy, see N. Hobbs, "Sources of Gain in Psychotherapy," *American Psychologist,* XVII (1962), 741-47.

haven. He would no doubt have responded to the attention he would get and doubtless would have become fluent fairly soon in the clinic atmosphere. However, an effective solution for the stuttering in these cases usually requires extensive psychotherapy, much more than most speech therapists can provide. These stutterers tend to need long-term psychotherapy of considerable depth. The majority are people with inadequately developed egos. For many of these cases, the cup of love and affection seems never to become filled. And, among the more severe ones, the clinical problem is further complicated by the feeling that any help they get is undeserved.

## SUMMARY

Perhaps, at this point, it would help if we present a summary chart of the distinguishing features for each of the patterns described.

FOUR COMMON PATTERNS OF CLINICAL PROBLEMS

| | | *Common and Prominent* | *Relatively Rare* |
|---|---|---|---|
| Pattern I | *Overt* | Devices to avoid, hide, disguise, deny, circumlocute. Ritualistic behavior; speech on residual air. | Long uninterrupted prolongations or repetitions or tremors. Facial contortions, "convulsive" movements. |
| | *Covert* | Embarrassment, shame, specific word fears, some guilt. | Frustration, anger, hostility. |
| Pattern II | *Overt* | Struggling, facial contortions, tremors, "convulsive" mannerisms, compulsive stuttering and talking. | Avoidance, postponement, disguise, giving up. |
| | *Covert* | Frustration, anger, aggression, some guilt. | Embarrassment, word or situation fears, anxiety. |
| Pattern III | *Overt* | Hesitancy, retrials, halfhearted attempts, abulia. | Struggle, severe contortions or tremors, disguise, rituals. |
| | *Covert* | Anxiety, frustration. | Hostility, guilt. |
| Pattern IV | *Overt* | Weak speech attempts, extended prolongations or silent blocks, abulia. | Aggressive speech attempts, struggle, tremors, facial contortions. |

FOUR COMMON PATTERNS OF CLINICAL PROBLEMS

| | *Common and Prominent* | *Relatively Rare* |
|---|---|---|
| *Covert* | Impotence, helplessness, frustration, low ego strength, guilt, anxiety, suggestibility. | Outwardly expressed hostility. |

In conclusion, secondary stuttering as a clinical problem is difficult to comprehend. It is much like Robert Frost's America (*12*:20-24):

. . . It can't be seen from the outside
Or inside either for that matter. . . .

The identification of chronic, disordered fluency as confirmed stuttering tells us too little about an individual's problem. We must identify the other features of the problem stuttering currently represents in each case and evaluate their significance for therapy. There are many possible features and innumerable combinations. No two stutterers can be expected to present the same pattern. However, this does not mean that effective help for these people requires a separate and distinct treatment for each and every case. Certain features are shared to some extent by nearly all cases and may respond to common approaches. In addition, many cases present patterns of clinically significant features sufficiently similar to indicate common therapy needs. We have presented four such patterns encountered frequently during the course of our own clinical practice. There are others. When a secondary stutterer comes to us for help, we ask ourselves this question, "What *kind* of problem does this particular stutterer have?" Only by identifying the individual features and discerning their relative significance for therapy can we hope to provide a solution for an encouraging percentage of these secondary stutterers that has some satisfying permanence.

IN PRECEDING CHAPTERS, INFORMATION HAS BEEN PRESENTED about the beginnings of stuttering, about its course of development into a full-blown problem, and about the clinical significance of the numerous and varied features that may constitute stuttering in the confirmed stage. Suggested references have provided information about the many different approaches and techniques useful in the treatment of this disorder. In this final chapter, we concern ourselves with the *prevention* of stuttering.

# 5 prevention

## LIMITATIONS

Let us first discuss certain aspccts of stuttering which we probably cannot expect to prevent. There are two. One is the broken speech from which clinical problems of stuttering usually emerge. There are three principal reasons why children cannot be expected to talk without periodically exhibiting unusual amounts of fluency disruptions. First, breaks in the fluency of oral communication are too much of an integral part of normal development and normal speech. Secondly, there is a definite tendency, in the American culture at least, to put a premium on the early establishment of many developmental skills, including those connected with communication. Though the majority of children may respond to such demands without appreciable adverse consequences of any kind, some cannot, and a percentage of these children will tend to reveal their inadequacies in occasional flurries of fragmented sentences and words. Lastly, there is sufficient evidence to indicate that a few children, by virtue of their unique inheritance, are destined to be unable to avoid intermittent occurrences of excessive amounts of broken speech.

The other aspect of stuttering that cannot be prevented, at least in some cases, is the appearance of advanced signs of the disorder. Some children react very early to the occurrence of fluency breaks in their speech. And among others whose stuttering begins later, there are those who seem to have very low tolerances for sensed interruptions in the utterance of words.

## General approach to preventive measures

What we do believe can be prevented, in the great majority of instances, is the establishment of stuttering as a complicated clinical problem. As we pointed out earlier, this occurs when feelings of concern or frustration become sufficiently intense to cause a child to feel that the periodic difficulty he has in talking is insoluble. Emotional reactions are internalized, behavior patterns become self-reinforcing, and the stuttering then becomes difficult if not impossible to eradicate. We believe there would be few cases of secondary stuttering if early forms of broken speech or initial signs of advanced stuttering can be prevented from becoming the focus of pronounced feelings of concern.

Unfortunately, particularly for the beginning therapist, there is no single, simple way of accomplishing this. Informing parents and teachers about the evil consequences of adverse listener reactions to broken speech helps a great deal, but it is not enough in many instances. We must be prepared to recognize other factors in a child or his environment which are responsible for the precipitation or the aggravation of beginning stuttering. In addition, the speech therapist must be skilled in ways of educating and counseling parents, and, when necessary, must know how to work directly with children for preventive purposes.

Identification of individual needs for effective prevention is the first important requisite. Children who may be in danger of acquiring clinical disorders of stuttering vary in the problems requiring attention in much the same way that secondary stutterers do. There are significant patterns of different conditions and circumstances among these people just as there are for the confirmed stutterers. And the possibilities for combinations of factors also are numerous. However, clinical experience has led us to conclude that the situation is similar to that for secondary stutterers, i.e., certain relatively distinct patterns occur frequently. Hence, successful prevention in many instances may be accomplished by similar approaches. Again, to provide information about the patterns we find are presented most frequently, we shall cite some illustrative cases.

### *Sandy*

This boy began to stutter quite suddenly about a month after the beginning of his second school year. The interruptions consisted of frequent, excessive series of initial syllables and single word repetitions. He occasionally appeared frustrated in his efforts to talk, but there was no evidence of concern, and most of the time he seemed unaware of the breaks in his speech. The parents were unable to explain the behavior. So far as they knew, Sandy was an unusually healthy child, emotionally as well as physically. Developmental skills during the preschool years had occurred, if anything, somewhat in advance of normative standards. He had talked early and always had been a very verbal child. He had not been a difficult child to discipline. Information from the parent interviews indicated no more than a normal amount of intrafamily stress and strife. Both parents were college graduates who felt they had been succeeding fairly well in raising their daughter and two sons sensibly in relation to current ideas about child rearing. About the only special trouble Sandy had presented was a problem of keeping him occupied and answering all his questions. He seemed to have more curiosity than most children.

He had been eager to start school and had adjusted well to that situation the first year. At the beginning of the second year, he had been placed in an enriched program which he appeared to enjoy very much. He talked daily about the interesting things done or seen at school. He presented a picture of a stable, well adjusted, contented child. The parents had explored the only explanation they thought made any sense—some dire traumatic experience that Sandy couldn't tell them about. They had visions of his having been the victim of some sex pervert. They reviewed events of the past week, they talked with neighbors, they visited his teacher. Nothing that would explain the trouble was discovered.

The stuttering continued on into the second week. Signs were beginning to develop suggesting that Sandy was reacting at times to the broken fluency. He would start a questioning sentence, then interrupt it with, "Oh, never mind." The explanation came suddenly one night when the father overheard his son's bedtime prayer. It ended with, "And please, God, help me to get all my schoolwork done." The next day, the incident was discussed with the boy's teacher. She made some immediate changes in his school program. The stuttering began to subside in just a few days, and it disappeared completely in about three weeks.

Except for the abrupt onset and the fact that the explanation was less obvious at first than it is in most instances, this case was almost classic in its clarity as one of the frequent patterns found among beginning stutterers. The interruptions, though normal in form, exceeded normalcy in amounts and in frequency. The child involved was a bright, healthy, precocious youngster. He lived in an essentially healthy home environment. The parents were well educated and, economically and socially, they were representative of the upper middle class. We find many children with similar personal characteristics and family backgrounds where beginning stuttering is related to stress associated with a drive to excel. In addition to the

56 See "The Demosthenes Complex," in *Stuttering*, ed. D. A. Barbara (New York: Julian Press, 1954), Chapter 6.

features found in Sandy, many of these children are said by their parents to be high-strung, nervous, excitable, sensitive, or perhaps "hyper." They tend to be highly competitive, and frequently are among the overachievers in school. They often are described as children who "talk too fast," and some parents or teachers will add, "and too much."

### *Basic Treatment Needs*

The general approach to preventive measures for children in this group should be fairly obvious. They do not need speech work, as such. Indeed, directing the attentions of these children to their speech by suggesting they slow down or modify their manner of talking in some other way is likely to be ineffective; in fact, such procedures would carry the great risk of precipitating the very thing treatment, if possible, must prevent: the creation of concern about the broken speech.

The most suitable approach for these and for most cases of beginning stuttering is *indirect.* The children should not be made to realize that their speech is the source of any parental or professional concern or the target of any treatment. What is needed in each instance is the elimination or at least considerable alleviation of the source of the stress which is serving to precipitate the excessive disfluency. Changes must be effected in the conditions or circumstances that are causing the individual to strive so mightily, to be so competitive, to always be trying to do very well. Some of these children, because of their precociousness, seldom have experienced anything but approval for their behavior. They understandably seek to maintain that pleasant status. Others appear to have absorbed the idea of doing one's best from family attitudes. And, sometimes, we find children in this group who are being driven beyond their capabilities by parents who are trying to satisfy their own emotional needs through the achievements of the children.

Preventive treatment for these cases obviously is most effectively carried out through parents or other close associates. Sometimes all that is necessary is some discussion of the problems supplemented by suggested reading.

**57** Useful books and pamphlets for this purpose include:

W. Johnson, *An Open Letter to the Mother of a Stuttering Child* (Danville, Ill.: Interstate Printers and Publishers, 1941).

C. Van Riper, *Teaching Your Child to Talk* (New York: Harper & Row, Publishers, Inc., 1950).

C. Miller, *Is Your Child Beginning to Stutter?* (Danville, Ill.: Interstate Printers and Publishers, 1960).

M. Fraser, (Publisher), *Stuttering: Its Prevention* (Memphis, Tenn.: Speech Foundation of America, 1962).

F. Robinson, *Children Who Stutter* (Oxford, O.: Miami University Speech-Hearing Clinic, 1955).

W. Johnson, *Stuttering and What You Can Do About It* (Minneapolis: University of Minnesota Press, 1961).

*R.Mulder, Tangled Tongues: Helping the Stuttering Child* (Monmouth, Ore.: Oregon College of Education, 1960).

Any recommended reading, of course, must be carefully selected by the therapist for its suitability in terms of the reader's educational background and his emotional relationship to the child. We must be particularly careful of the possibility that unexplained reading material may create or aggravate harmful guilt feelings.

### Parent counseling

In other cases, preventive measures must consist of counseling procedures involving a series of meetings. The basic aims of such counseling "interviews" are to (*a*) obtain additional information about a child's environment and his beginning stuttering, (*b*) provide education about speech development and stuttering, (*c*) allow parents to verbalize attitudes and feelings about their child's behavior, (*d*) help them understand the circumstances associated with the broken speech, and (*e*) to provide a setting in which parents themselves may arrive at appropriate steps to be taken or be receptive to the therapist's suggestions.

58 For more detailed information about counseling procedures, see:

A. T. Murphy and R. M. Fitzsimons, *Stuttering and Personality Dynamics* (New York: Ronald Press, 1960), Chapter 12.

Z. S. Wolpe, "Play Therapy, Psychodrama, and Parent Counseling," in *Handbook of Speech Pathology,* ed. L. E. Travis (New York: Appleton-Century-Crofts, Inc., 1957), 1015-23.

B. Bettelheim, *Dialogues with Mothers* (New York: Glencoe, 1962).

H. L. Luper and R. L. Mulder, *Stuttering: Therapy for Children* (Englewood Cliffs, N. J.: Prentice-Hall, Inc., 1964), Chapter 3.

*Harvey*

A local public-school therapist on her first job after graduation introduced us to Harvey. She called to ask if we would see a boy and perhaps tell her what she should do. We asked what the problem seemed to be and she told us,

> "Well, it's a little boy in the first grade. He has a severe articulation disorder and also a problem with language. He still says things like "me dood it" or "her went away." His mother told me that he was very late in talking. She said they had him checked twice by physicians because of his speech. Both doctors told the parents there was nothing wrong with the boy and that he probably would outgrow the trouble. He's almost seven now. He hasn't done well in school this year. His teacher said she thought they shouldn't pass him, although he had a score of 102 on a Stanford-Binet. He has responded to work on the articulation. I've worked on three sounds this year, the *f*, the *k*, and the [θ]. But he still has a long way to go. He has trouble with *s* and [ʃ] and [tʃ] and the *l* and *r*. There are also some vowel sounds that he doesn't pronounce clearly."
>
> "Sounds like delayed speech and articulation, sure enough. What's the problem? Does the mother want you to talk the teacher into passing the child?"
>
> "No, it's not that. He has begun to stutter. I've been noticing it now for about a month and I think it's getting worse. I've never said anything about it and the parents haven't either. I'm afraid it's all this work on the speech that's causing it. He works awful hard for me. I thought maybe I should stop the work, but he needs so much help."
>
> "All right, bring him in this Saturday morning and we'll take a look at him. Can you tell him that you are coming in to visit and just invite him to come along? Then we won't be taking so much of a chance that he might become more concerned about his speech than he already may be."

On Saturday morning, we introduced Harvey to one of the senior student therapists who had been carefully instructed to "examine" the boy in a very casual and informal way while showing him around the clinic and exploring the playroom. As we watched and listened through a two-way mirror, I verbalized my observations and impressions for the therapist's benefit as well as for my own.

"Yeah, there's some possible signs of stuttering, all right. . . . There's all those repetitions and there are some prolongations, too. . . . But notice that faltering and fumbling he does as he talks. Listen now as he's telling Janey about his Dad's boat . . . at least, I think that's what he's talking about. . . . He talks in spurts. . . . He says, 'My . . my . . . my Dad, him dot . . . . him . . . him dot dit . . . . . dit . . . dit . . . him dot dit boat . . . bid boat.' . . . He seems to be groping for the words and the ways to put them together. . . . This looks like a good case of an unorganized language system. . . . The articulation problem is there, sure enough, but I'm inclined to believe that the more critical problem right now is the language deficiency. Harvey appears to be one of those poorly organized children that Bluemel has described so well. You remarked about his poor motor coordination. These children usually reveal evidence of a delay or deficiency in several motor and sensory areas. . . . But the *thinking* of these children seems poorly developed, too. . . . Maybe it is basically a delay in auditory perceptual development. . . . They often mispronounce as well as misarticulate words. . . . Many of these children become clutterers before developing obvious signs of stuttering. And that may be what this boy is. His rate of broken speech doesn't suggest cluttering at the moment, but Weiss (Search Item No. 15), in his most recent book, you know, claims that cluttering may occur at slow rates in some instances. He would no doubt diagnose this boy's problems as cluttering. . . . In either case, it's more of a language than a speech problem."

"Should I stop working on the articulation?"

"Probably, at least for awhile. But we've seen enough here. Let's go back in the office to talk about treatment needs."

59 See C. S. Bluemel, *The Riddle of Stuttering* (Danville, Ill.: Interstate Publishing Co., 1957), Chapters 1, 2, and 3.

### *Basic Treatment Needs*

What we told our colleague was this, essentially: if we are to prevent children like Harvey from acquiring clinical problems of stuttering, we must help them get their language systems organized. Among other things, these children must be provided with simple models. Their comprehension usually is all right and what they try to do is to talk in the long sentences they hear all the time. But their unorganized systems, their neuromotor and perceptual deficiencies just won't allow them to do that. They must first have opportunities to establish less complicated language forms. Simple nursery rhymes are good for these children. We can have them memorize little pieces to speak. They have to catch on to the *idea* of language forms and units. Most children do this with very little assistance. Those like Harvey have to be helped with that in much the same way that a cerebral palsied child may need to work consciously to control his unruly muscles for breathing or walking.

We should have these children participate in unison talking. Good use can be made of the echo speech described by Van Riper (*37*:409). And, most importantly, we must not ignore the parents of these children. This can be a difficult problem for many of them to understand, since these children are so often physically healthy. All that seems to be wrong with them is their speech. Parents must understand. And much can be done in the home to supplement the work of the therapist, particularly by having parents respond to a child's fumbling efforts to talk with simply stated sentences said in casual, matter-of-fact ways. When a child like Harvey says something like, "Me think . . . . me . . . . me think . . . . Daddy . . time . . . Daddy . . Daddy time do . . . . do . . . do work," the mother should respond with, "Yes, it's time for Daddy to go to work." Other suggestions for the preventive treatment of these cases may be found in Bluemel's book (Search Item No. 59).

### *Laura*

A third *kind* of beginning stutterer may be illustrated by the story of Laura. We first saw her when she was just three-and-a-half years old. She had been stuttering for about four months. She repeated the first word of nearly every communication and sometimes of every sentence. She would say, "I . . . I . . . I . . . I . . I have a new dolly." She was the youngest of two children who were thirteen years apart in their ages. When Laura was conceived, her mother was just becoming freed of the time- and energy-consuming tasks related to the raising of her other child. She had become busy in many different social and community activities, and she was especially enjoying taking an active part in furthering her husband's political ambitions. He recently had become county prosecutor, wanted to become the state's attorney, and occasionally dreamed of living in the governor's house. He was a calm, easy-going man, but busy, busy, busy. Laura's mother was a frenetic individual who always looked busy and who got some of her greatest pleasures from compliments about her willingness to serve and her hard work on committees.

This was a good home. These parents loved both their children. Though Laura was something of a surprise and her mother said that she had some feelings of resentment during the pregnancy, it was an unusually easy birth, and the baby turned out to be very easy to take care of. And it became easy to have the babysitting done by the older daughter, though she resented it bitterly. She seldom paid much attention to her little sister in the daytime. The mother honestly enjoyed spending time with Laura, but there so often was not enough time to listen to her relate her experiences, to describe her activities, to tell of her troubles. The mother would say, "That's just fine, honey. You play in your room like a good little girl while I finish these telephone calls." The father often talked to her while he was reading a brief. Her sister would say, "Get lost."

We believe the stuttering in this case was clearly a sign of insecurity and uncertainty. This girl seldom knew whether she would be given time to talk. She doubtless felt in the way among such busy people who had so little time or apparent interest in her activities. There was marked ambivalence in her behavior around adults. We must remember that whenever we speak, we offer ourselves. And, if this offering is not acceptable, an essential insecurity results. Guilt feelings may also develop. Stutterers like Laura probably are good examples of Sheehan's (27:135) observations about primary guilt as a source of stuttering.

### *Basic Treatment Needs*

We find many beginning stutterers like Laura, children who live in worlds that continually foster approach-avoidance conflicts at the interpersonal relationship level. The specific patterns of circumstances are infinite in number and in their component features. But all are filled with anxiety and guilt-producing situations almost daily.

Preventing stuttering in these cases from growing into complex clinical problems is quite difficult at times. The stuttering label and similar harmful adverse listener reactions to the speech may be avoided, but it is not always so easy to implement other equally important preventive measures. It is the interpersonal relationship between the child and his parents that must be improved. The competition for his attention must be removed. He must be given his fair opportunity to talk and thus to establish a more acceptable self-concept.

*Environmental Manipulation*

Prevention may be accomplished in some of these cases by means of environmental changes. Sometimes the needed change can take place within the child's home. In Laura's case, for instance, we were able to impress the parents with the importance of immediate preventive measures (we did it by inviting them to attend a group meeting of adult stutterers), and they proceeded to find time to devote to their daughter. Few of these younger children are in need of the trained ear of the psychologist or the psychiatrist. The majority need only an attentive and interested listener long enough to establish some adequate feelings of security and self-esteem. It probably always is best if the listener is a child's own parent, but it need not be. In fact, it need not be a human. One of our professional colleagues prevented stuttering from becoming a clinical problem in one child by having the parents buy him a dog. He stopped stuttering within a month. When a child is hungry, it seems to make little difference who feeds him.

Sometimes the need for a more literal change of environment is indicated. We recall one case in which stuttering began in a three-year-old boy who had a five-year-old sister. The sister's language skills were unusually good, and she was also a very verbal child. She talked practically all of the time, as a matter of fact. As the boy's language became well enough established for frequent, practical use, he found himself too often unable to use it. His sister finished everything he started. This boy's stuttering subsided rapidly after the parents arranged for his sister to spend a few weekends with nearby relatives who had some young children. The boy never seemed to resent his sister's special privilege, probably because he had his parents' attentive ears all the time she was gone and was freed of frustrating interruptions.

Also, advantage may be taken of summer or weekend camps as a way of changing environments to effect the desired prevention. A major function of many camp counselors is the role of parent substitute. Their tolerant ears are always available. However, when such methods are utilized, their effectiveness may be temporary unless the home environment also is changed.

*Therapy*

Certain forms of therapy also are appropriate for some of these beginning stutterers. Though any of these thera-

60

Prepare a single paragraph description of each of the specific forms of applicable therapies found in these references:

R. F. Hejna, *Speech Disorders and Nondirective Therapy* (New York: Ronald Press, 1960), Chapters 4, 5, and 6.

A. T. Murphy and R. M. Fitzsimons, *Stuttering and Personality Dynamics* (New York: Ronald Press, 1960), Chapters 8, 9, and 10.

P. J. Glasner, "Psychotherapy of the Young Stutterer," in *The Psychotherapy of Stuttering*, ed. D. A. Barbara (Springfield, Ill.: C. C. Thomas, 1962), 250-56.

G. L. Wyatt and H. M. Herzan, "Therapy with Stuttering Children and Their Mothers," *American Journal of Orthopsychiatry*, XXXII (1962), 645-59.

pies may involve children directly in the treatment process, they must be thought of and utilized as *indirect* approaches for these cases. Beginning stutterers who are exposed to these forms of therapy must not be made aware that their speech is the target of the activity. This sometimes creates a special problem. A child who becomes curious about the reason for being included in such a program, even though it consists of play activities, may begin to wonder if it has something to do with his speech. This can be a particularly logical reaction if he discovers that the "teacher" is a speech therapist.

### *Gordon*

The next case, and the last in this section, actually is not an example of beginning stuttering so far as the fluency pattern was concerned. This boy's speech, as we shall see, was normal. However, he represents a fairly large group of children for whom preventive measures are indicated.

We learned about Gordon from the following letter:

Dear Sir:

Our son stutters sometimes. He is five years old and will be going to kindergarten this fall. We think he should have some help for his speech before he goes to school. We would like to enroll him in your summer clinic.

The following reply was sent:

Dear Mrs. ________:

Before we can enroll your son in our summer clinic, we first would need to see him, evaluate his problem, and then we can discuss his difficulty and our clinic program with you and your husband.

We could do that a week from this coming Saturday at 10:00 A.M. If this should be an inconvenient time, please let us know. Otherwise, we shall look forward to seeing you then.

In view of your son's age and the kind of problem he seems to have, may we suggest that you not tell him he is being brought to a Speech Clinic for an examination. Per-

> haps you can say that you and his father must come to Oxford to see a man and that he can come along for the ride. We have playroom facilities and, if it seems important to do so, we can examine him without having him be aware of our interest in his speech.

The suggested subterfuge, which we believe is important to suggest for any youngster about whose stuttering we cannot be certain before observation, turned out to be wise in this case. Our observations of Gordon, together with information from his parents, indicated that he was a normally healthy and intelligent youngster. Like many boys, his speech and language skills were not as well established by five as they had been for his sisters. However, he did not appear to be delayed in those areas. His articulation was good and his language was well on the way to becoming established. We observed this boy and listened to his speech at length. He did repeat words and phrases and, occasionally, an initial syllable, and he fumbled and hesitated at times. At one point, for example, as the staff therapist was keeping him occupied with a picture book, he said, "Yeah, I saw one like that in . . . . . in . . . in a . . . in a zoo. But . . . but that one was a . . . . . . was a . . . . . . well, was bigger and had a big horn on its face, like a . . . . . like a hippo . . . . . . hippotopamus. I can't say that word right."

All of his broken speech was of this variety. In every instance, it was related to his search for a word or to unsureness about pronunciation. His "stuttering," we felt certain, was a reflection of normal problems connected with the acquisition of his oral-communication system. Gordon had three older sisters, all of whom had talked very well by the fifth year. These parents had never seen much broken speech in their daughters. They were aware that boys generally are somewhat slower than girls in developing, but had not realized that this often included speech. They also had heard about stuttering and especially that it is more common among boys. Though they did not feel that their son's was a serious stuttering problem, they were sure that was what he was doing.

We asked what, if anything, had ever been said to Gordon about his speech. "Well, we tell him to slow down sometimes or to think about what he wants to say before he talks." We then asked if they ever referred to the interruptions as stuttering when they were talking to him. "Yes, sometimes. Just the other night at supper," his mother said, "I remember saying 'You're stuttering again. Try to think of the word before you say it.'"

These parents were fortunate. We saw no signs in this boy of any concern about his speech. *Stuttering*, to him, obviously had no unpleasant significance. We concluded that the reason lay in the general emotional climate of this home and that, although the parents wanted their son to stop stuttering, they had not used the word or reacted in any other way that would suggest to him that he was doing something that distressed his parents or was "bad."

### *Basic Treatment Needs*

Preventive measures for stutterers like Gordon may require nothing more complicated than parent education. Among the things we must help parents of these children understand, of course, is the harmful consequences of adverse listener reactions. These must be explained in ways that avoid the generation of any guilt feelings. When parents of such a case express the thought that they have been "doing all the wrong things" and are distressed, we try to reassure them by relating a fact: no parents ever raised a child without making mistakes occasionally.

Information about the development of speech should be provided at an understandable level. The child's general development needs to be discussed along with any special problems in addition to the speech. Informative pamphlets or books such as those listed in Search Item No. 57 may be supplied or suggested. It is important with these cases to actively encourage parents to contact the therapist if the broken speech should happen to become more frequent and/or excessive or to change noticeably in form. Many parents who have been assured about the normalcy of their children's speech are reluctant to risk being told a second time that there is nothing to be concerned about. If the therapist does not hear from the parents of one of these children, it is advisable to contact them after a month or so. Even when there has been no further cause for concern, the parents thus will be assured of the therapist's continued interest.

## Preventive treatment for the advanced stutterer

When we are confronted with a child who has gone beyond the beginning stage, one who presents an advanced pattern of stuttering behavior, it still is possible to have him succeed in avoiding the establishment of stuttering as a complex clinical problem. Preventive approaches for these children are of two types, *indirect* and *direct*.

### *Indirect*

Methods representative of the indirect approach have already been discussed. Any of them may be used successfully with cases of advanced stuttering. As we pointed out earlier, the effects of concern and frustration are usually gradual. Stuttering seldom changes abruptly from the beginning signs into the secondary stage. And if we have the opportunity to treat a child fairly early in the course of the stuttering development, indirect methods should be the preferred choice. If the circumstances responsible for the aggravation of the stuttering together with other possible factors related to its onset can be removed, the difficulty may be resolved without the child having to become involved directly in any treatment.

### *Direct*

The term *direct* in this context implies not only that the child is involved directly in treatment, but that he is presumed to be fully aware of the purpose of treatment. He knows that his stuttering is the reason for his visits to a clinic or his enrollment in any other treatment program. Thus, when some direct method is to be applied, it is assumed that an indirect method no longer would be effective or possibly practicable.

#### *Criteria for the Decision to Use Direct Methods*

The decision about the appropriateness or the necessity for utilizing a direct method for preventive purposes rests on the therapist's judgment. The following are three criteria that may be utilized in helping with the decision:

1. The severity and complexity of the stuttering behavior. The early advanced stuttering of some children is characterized by considerable struggle and literal difficulty in uttering words at times. These children often cannot avoid becoming secondary stutterers unless they can be helped in finding a less troublesome way of uttering those words.

2. The degree of emotional involvement. Among the young advanced stutterers, this factor ranges from a slight amount to intense distress. It usually is possible to make a fairly accurate judgment by observing a child's general behavior in speaking situations and particularly the extent to which he is inclined to avoid answering questions after rapport has been established. A child may do little obvious stuttering, yet be well on his way to becoming a confirmed stutterer.
3. Parental cooperation factor. Some children, who otherwise could be helped by some indirect method, must be exposed to direct treatment because the parents are unable or possibly unwilling to cooperate in a preventive program. With these children, we must risk the possibility that a direct approach may generate more harmful amounts of concern.

### *Factors Related to Prognosis*

In addition to deciding that a child must have some direct help if he is to avoid the secondary stage of stuttering, there are certain factors to be considered in connection with the probable success of the preventive treatment. One of these is suggested by the third item above, the parental cooperation factor. The encouraging results a child may achieve in the therapy session may be completely canceled by the home environment. It is very difficult to save some children from the emotional damage inflicted by parents. We must try, but we also must be realistic.

Another factor related to a favorable program for prevention is intelligence. Generally, children with higher intelligence respond better to direct treatment. There are things children must understand and be able to learn if we are to help them. However, some children whose IQ's place them in the dull normal group respond very well to direct methods. They may not understand what they learn, but they may take and follow simple directions very well.

A third factor of importance to prognosis is the presence of other problems which may be competing with the stuttering for the child's attention and time. A child may be highly interested in having help for his stuttering, but, at the same time, he may be equally interested in or concerned about his school grades, his hobby, his cub scout activities, or any of many other possible areas of interest or anxiety.

### *Direct Treatment Methods*

What individual children in this group may need in the way of direct help for their growing stuttering problem depends on the pattern of the stuttering behavior. Generally, we find that they fall into two broad groups. Those in one group are the children who are reacting to their developing feelings of concern or frustration by more or less compulsive struggle behavior. We must help these cases find easier ways of talking. Van Riper (*38*:376) provides a pertinent example:

"THERAPIST. I understand that you've been having a lot of trouble talking lately, Peter.

PETER. Yea, I, I, I, I've been ssssss . . . . . . . stutt . . . . stuttering. (The boy squeezed his eyes shut and fast tremors appeared on his tightly closed lips. The word finally emerged after a surge of tension and a head jerk.) I've been stuttering bad.

THERAPIST. So I see. Let's try to help you. I know what you're doing wrong. You're fighting yourself. You're pushing too hard. Let me show you how you just stuttered and then show you how to do it easy. (Therapist demonstrates.)

PETER. Oh!

THERAPIST. Now I'm going to ask you a question and if you stutter while answering it, I'll join you but show you how to let it come out easy. OK? All right, how close is the nearest drugstore to your house?

PETER. It's over on the next b . . . b . . . bbbbbbblock. (While the boy is struggling, the therapist first duplicates what he is doing, and then slowly slides out of the fixation without tension. The child hears him, opens his eyes to watch him, and an expression of surprise is seen on the child's face.)

THERAPIST. Yea, I told you I was going to stutter right along with you but you'll have to watch me, if you're going to learn how to let the words come out easy. Let's try another. If I went through the front door of your house, how would I find your room?

PETER. YYYYYYYYYYou'd . . . (The child joined the therapist in his grin.) Yyyou'd have to ggggggo upstairs.

THERAPIST. That second time you didn't push it so hard, did you. Good. You went like this . . . (Therapist demonstrates.) Look, you've got to learn how to stutter my way, nice and easy, either like th-th-th-this or like th . . . is. (Therapist prolongs the sound easily and without effort.) Now let's play a speech game of follow the leader. You be my echo and say just what I say and stutter just like I do. Sometimes I'll stutter your way and sometimes my way, the better way, the way you've got to learn to do it."

Those in the other group are the ones who are trying to solve their felt problem by not talking any more than they have to. Speech to them is becoming painful, threatening, for they fear the consequences of talking. These children must be helped to discover that talking can be not only possible but enjoyable. Sing songs perhaps as a start. Read poems together. Puppets are frequently very good. The children forget themselves and their fear of talking. When they have become more willing to talk, take turns telling stories. Another possibility is to have a child narrate television commercials with the volume turned down. Filmstrips of cowboy stories and cartoons may be used in the same way. Other suggestive methods for helping these children lose their growing fear of talking may be found in the book by Luper and Mulder (Search Item No. 58).

## Summary and conclusion

Secondary stuttering is easier to prevent than to treat. The difficulty can be impossible to eliminate once the advanced patterns of behavior become fixed and self-perpetuating. However, if stuttering can be treated before that occurs, many children can avoid years of social misery and economic penalties. Preventive measures have been described. A number of cases have been presented to illustrate the common patterns found among young stutterers. There are others. And there are patterns within patterns. But similar prominent features are to be found in many cases. Differences must be considered, but similarities allow common approaches to be applied. We cannot hope to save every youngster from becoming a secondary stutterer. But careful case study, the application of acquired skill in discerning the significant features, and the effective use of the appropriate preventive treatment can save the majority.

# *bibliography*


1. Abbott, J. A., "Repressed Hostility as a Factor in Adult Stuttering," *Journal of Speech Disorders,* XII (1947).
2. Barbara, D., *Stuttering* (New York: Julian Press, 1954).
3. Berry, M. and J. Eisenson, *Speech Disorders* (New York: Appleton-Century-Crofts, Inc., 1956).
4. Bloodstein, O., "The Development of Stuttering: 1. Changes in Nine Basic Features," *Journal of Speech and Hearing Disorders,* XXV (1960).
5. Bluemel, C. S., "Primary and Secondary Stuttering," *Proceedings of the American Speech Correction Association* (1943).
6. ———, *The Riddle of Stuttering* (Danville, Ill.: The Interstate Printers & Publishers, Inc., 1957).
7. Eisenson, J., "A Perseverative Theory of Stuttering," in *Stuttering: A Symposium,* ed. J. Eisenson (New York: Harper & Row, Publishers, Inc., 1958).

8. Fraser, M. (Publisher), *Stuttering: Its Prevention* (Memphis, Tenn.: Speech Foundation of America, 1962).
9. Freed, G. H., *Anti-Stammering Device.* U.S. Patent Office, No. 2,818,065, Dec. 31, 1957.
10. Freund, H., "Psychopathological Aspects of Stuttering," *American Journal of Psychotherapy,* VII (1953).
11. Froeschels, E., "A Study of the Symptomatology of Stuttering," *Monatschrift fur Ohrenheil,* LV (1921).
12. Frost, R., "America Is Hard to See," from *In The Clearing* (New York: Holt, Rinehart and Winston, Inc., 1962).
13. Glauber, I. P., "The Psychoanalysis of Stuttering," in *Stuttering: A Symposium,* ed. J. Eisenson (New York: Harper & Row, Publishers, Inc., 1958).
14. Johnson, W., S. F. Brown, J. F. Curtis, C. W. Edney, and J. Keaster, *Speech Handicapped School Children* rev. ed. (New York: Harper & Row, Publishers, Inc., 1956).
15. Karlin, I. W., "A Psychosomatic Theory of Stuttering," *Journal of Speech Disorders,* XII (1947).
16. ———, "Stuttering: Basically an Organic Disorder," *Logos,* II (1959).
17. Klencke, H., *Die Heilung des Stotterns* (Leipzig: C. E. Kollman, 1862).
18. Klingbeil, G. M., "The Historical Background of the Modern Speech Clinic," *Journal of Speech Disorders,* IV (1939).
19. Lee, B. S., "Artificial Stutter," *Journal of Speech and Hearing Disorders,* XVI (1951).
20. Miller, N. E., "Experimental Studies of Conflict," in *Personality and the Behavior Disorders,* ed. J. McV. Hunt (New York: Ronald Press, 1944).
21. Moncur, J. P., "Parental Domination in Stuttering," *Journal of Speech and Hearing Disorders,* XVII (1952).
22. Murphy, A. T. and R. M. Fitzsimons, *Stuttering and Personality Dynamics* (New York: Ronald Press, 1960).
23. Mysak, E. C., "Servo Theory and Stuttering," *Journal of Speech and Hearing Disorders,* XXV (1960).
24. Neeley, J. N., "A Study of the Speech Behavior of Stutterers and Nonstutterers Under Normal and Delayed Auditory Feedback," *Journal of Speech and Hearing Disorders,* Monograph Supplement No. 7, 1961.

25. Orton, S., *Reading, Writing, and Speech Problems in Children* (New York: W. W. Norton and Co., 1937).
26. Peters, R. W., "The Effect of Changes in Side-Tone Delay and Level upon Rate of Oral Reading of Normal Speakers," *Journal of Speech and Hearing Disorders,* XIX (1954).
27. Sheehan, J., "Conflict Theory of Stuttering," in *Stuttering: A Symposium,* ed. J. Eisenson (New York: Harper & Row, Publishers, Inc., 1958).
28. Smith, K. U., *Delayed Sensory Feedback and Behavior* (Philadelphia: W. B. Saunders Co., 1962).
29. Ssikorski, J. A., *Ueber das Stottern* (Berlin: A. Hirschwald, 1891).
30. Stromsta, C., "A Methodology Related to the Determination of the Phase Angle of Bone-Conducted Speech Sound Energy of Stutterers and Non-Stutterers." Unpublished dissertation, The Ohio State University, 1956.
31. ———, "Experimental Blockage of Phonation by Distorted Side-Tone," *Journal of Speech and Hearing Research,* II (1959).
32. Sullivan, H. S., *The Interpersonal Theory of Psychiatry* (New York: W. W. Norton and Co., 1953).
33. ———, *The Psychiatric Interview* (New York: W. W. Norton and Co., 1954).
34. Tomatis, A., "Relations entre l'Audition et la Phonation," *Extroit des Annales des Telecommunications,* Tome II, (1956).
35. Travis, L. E., "My Present Thinking on Stuttering," *Western Speech,* X (1946).
36. ———, *Speech Pathology* (New York: Appleton-Century-Crofts, Inc., 1931).
37. ———, "The Unspeakable Feelings of People with Special Reference to Stuttering," in *Handbook of Speech Pathology,* ed. L. E. Travis (New York: Appleton-Century-Crofts, Inc., 1957).
38. Van Riper, C., *Speech Correction,* 4th ed. (Englewood Cliffs, N. J.: Prentice-Hall, Inc., 1963).
39. Weiss, D. A., "Therapy of Cluttering," *Folia Phoniatrica,* XII (1960).
40. West, R., "An Agnostic's Speculations about Stuttering,"

in *Stuttering: A Symposium,* ed. J. Eisenson (New York: Harper & Row, Publishers, Inc., 1958).
41. ———, L. Kennedy, and A. Carr, *The Rehabilitation of Speech* (New York: Harper & Row, Publishers, Inc., 1937).
42. Wyllie, J., *The Disorders of Speech* (Edinburgh: Oliver and Boyd, 1894).

# *index*

# *index*